Arthritis

300 TIPS
for Making Life Easier

Arthritis

300 TIPS
for Making Life Easier

Shelley Peterman Schwarz

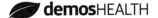

demosHEALTH

Visit our web site at www.demosmedpub.com

Library of Congress Cataloging-in-Publication Data

Schwarz, Shelley Peterman.
    Arthritis : 300 and more tips for making life easier / Shelley Peterman Schwarz.
      p. cm.
    Includes index.
    ISBN-13: 978-1-932603-67-5 (pbk. : alk. paper)
    ISBN-10:   1-932603-67-0 (pbk. : alk. paper)
    1. Arthritis—Popular works.   I. Title.
    RC933.S294   2009
    616.7'22—dc22   2008017418

Special discounts on bulk quantities of Demos Medical Publishing books are available to corporations, professional associations, pharmaceutical companies, health care organizations, and other qualifying groups. For details, please contact:

Special Sales Department
Demos Medical Publishing
386 Park Avenue South, Suite 301
New York, NY 10016
Phone: 800–532–8663 or 212–683–0072
Fax: 212–683–0118
E-mail: orderdept@demosmedpub.com

Printed in the United States of America
8   9   10   11   5   4   3   2   1

Contents

A Word from the Author

Dear Reader,

When I was diagnosed with multiple sclerosis (MS), in 1979, it changed my life in ways I could never imagine. For a few years, I tried to ignore the disease and pass as normal, but eventually my limitations became more serious and I began using a three-wheeled Amigo scooter to get around. It was then that I had to come to terms with the fact that I had a progressively degenerative disease that was having an impact on my life and the lives of my family and friends as well.

Because I am severely disabled by my chronic illness, I have had to modify, streamline, and make changes to the way I live. Over the years, I've learned some basic concepts that have helped me immensely, and I've learned thousands of simple time- and energy-saving tips that make a big difference in the quality of my life.

To update this book, I used my personal experience, my professional training as a teacher of the Deaf, and interviews I conducted with people living with arthritis and related medical conditions like fibromyalgia, lupus, osteoporosis, ankylosing spondylitis, and others. Talking to others with chronic illnesses and disabilities has taught me a lot about survival and the human spirit, and how strong and resilient people can be. We may not have a choice about having an illness, but we do have a choice in the way we react to it.

This book features tips to help you streamline daily activities, find ways to stay involved and in touch, and discover local, state, and national resources to make your life easier. The book is arranged in categories of daily activities for easy reference. At the beginning of each chapter, I share some of the insights and observations people have shared with me about living with arthritis. It is my hope that these simple, inexpensive hints will save you time and energy, lessen your frustration, and promote safety and independence.

In this book, I've tried to select the very best and most helpful resources for people living with arthritis and related medical conditions. Most of the products I mention in this book are available in drug, discount, hardware, building supply, and home improvement stores. A resource section at the end of each chapter will help you find the unique items you feel would be most helpful to you.

Keep in mind that product offerings change from time to time. If you have difficulty locating an item at the resource listed, do an Internet search on the term, and you will likely find an alternative source. If you still do not find what you are looking for, check with your doctor, clinic, or local arthritis support chapter for advice on products to meet your specific needs. I hope that learning how other people deal with the challenges of arthritis will help you keep a positive attitude on your journey. May my book inspire you and help you face the future with a sense of empowerment and control over your illness.

I wish you all the best,
Shelley Peterman Schwarz

P.S. If, after reading this book, you'd like to share your own **Tips for Making Life Easier**™, or if you just want to "chat" visit my web site, www.MakingLifeEasier.com or e-mail Shelley@MakingLifeEasier.com.

Acknowledgments

To my parents, Ruth and Bill Peterman who loved me unconditionally and taught me to believe in myself.

To my wonderful husband David, our daughter Jamie and son Andrew, who have been on this journey with me. Thank you for loving me even when I didn't love myself and for allowing me to find my own way in my own time. To David and Ronit, who have joined our family; I feel blessed to have you in my life. To my entire family, you fill my heart to overflowing.

To my friends and neighbors who have held my hand along the way, especially Judy Ross. I would have been lost without you. Thank you seems so inadequate.

To my amazing and talented assistant, Deborah Proctor, who also lives with significant disabilities. You are my right hand, in every sense of the word. We make quite a team! This journey I'm on and the work I do has been even more healing and rewarding because you are there with me.

CHAPTER 1

Basic Concepts for Making Life Easier

When you have arthritis, or any of over 100 arthritis-related conditions such as fibromyalgia, lupus, osteoporosis, ankylosing spondylitis, or bursitis, daily life can be filled with challenges. Activities you once took for granted—driving the car, doing the laundry, fixing meals, climbing stairs—can be difficult and painful. You may feel tired, stressed, depressed, and even angry at the pain and your inability to do the things you want to do.

Coping with any type of chronic condition means living in a world of never-ending change as symptoms flare up and then subside, often for no apparent reason. Some people find it easier to cope than others. I've learned from personal experience and from people with arthritis that tips and strategies to improve your attitude and mind set can be very helpful.

I hope you find these insights and observations that I hope will help you live a happier and more satisfying life.

1. **Look for ways to reduce your stress level and put yourself and your needs first.** This is not selfish or self-centered. You must take care of YOU first! You are the authority regarding your own body. Rest when you're tired. Be protective about how you spend your time and energy. Understand that day-to-day living uses a great deal of physical energy and there is an emotional and mental component to coping and adapting. Do the things that are important to you and your family. Give

yourself permission to say "No," without feeling guilty. When you are feeling better, you can say "Yes."

2. **Try not to be self-conscious about the visible symptoms of your arthritis.** It may be challenging, but look for ways to work around your problems. If you are self-conscious about the way you walk or need extra support when walking, loop your arm through your spouse's or friend's arm. Use a wheelchair if distances are too far to walk. (You could be recovering from surgery, a car accident, or a sports injury for all anyone knows.) If your hands are weak, ask the waitress at a restaurant to cut up your food in the kitchen before she brings it to the table. If you have trouble getting books off the shelf at the library or bookstore, see if a friend or an employee can accompany and help you. Don't let your visible (or invisible, for that matter) symptoms diminish your enjoyment when getting out. Family and friends want you to participate and live a full life.

3. **Keep your sense of humor!** Having trouble moving as fast as you used to, giving up a favorite activity like golf, or using a handicapped parking placard when you shop are not particularly funny. However, putting a humorous spin on everyday observations and situations breaks the tension and puts your problems in perspective. For example, if you drop or spill something and make a mess, say, "I learned this from my children." If you need to lean on someone to get from here to there, tease that some people will do anything for a little extra attention. If you are embarrassed by the orthopedic shoes you must wear, tell friends you're trying to set a new fashion trend. (And, why not? Who would have thought that platform shoes and spiked heels with pointed toes would be a fad?) Laughter is a great stress reducer.

4. **Surround yourself with caring, loving, and nurturing family members, friends, neighbors, and co-workers.** Give yourself permission to eliminate people and activities that drain your energy. If you're having a bad day, be honest with your family and friends. Explain that you may feel terrible in the morning but fine in the afternoon. Don't expect people to know what you are feeling unless you tell them.

5. **Tell people about your illness.** At any age, it can be difficult to share your feelings with your friends; it can be especially difficult if you're diagnosed with arthritis when you're young. Your friends may not know what having arthritis is really like for you. And they may not know what to say or do—so tell them. Also, tell your hair stylist, dentist, and customer-service people (as appropriate) that you may need their help.

6. **Keep a positive attitude**, even though it can be extremely difficult as your symptoms change, and the effectiveness of medications plays havoc with your life. It's perfectly natural to mourn the loss of function and independence for a brief time, but try not to get stuck there and wallow in self-pity or isolate yourself from the people who care about you.

7. **Deal with depression.** If you experience any combination of these symptoms—loss of appetite, feelings of sadness, difficulty sleeping, loss of your sense of humor, a sense of hopelessness, melancholy, or a "who cares" attitude—you are probably suffering from clinical depression. Please! Tell your doctor!!!

    Even though you have every right to be depressed about your diagnosis, depression is a treatable condition. A combination of antidepressants and/or psychotherapy can help lift your spirits and give you renewed energy to keep that all-important positive attitude.

8. **Remember: Your family and friends are not trained professionals.** In fact, they may also be hurting because of your diagnosis. Perhaps they, too, could benefit from talking to someone about their fears and frustrations.

9. **Listen to audiotapes, podcasts, and/or read books that promote positive thinking and deliver a healing message.** The public library and book stores offer an array of these materials. Tune into the free, weekly Internet radio program, Making Life Easier, at www.Making LifeEasier.com, to hear what others have learned about living with chronic illness that has helped them heal and move forward.

10. **Set priorities and focus on tasks that must be done.** Tackle one job at a time. Break down activities into a series of smaller steps and ask others to assist you with the difficult portions of the task. Avoid working or sitting for long periods in the same position. Move around periodically.

11. **Allow extra time to do everything** from eating, drinking, and dressing to walking, and writing. Recognize that everything takes longer when you have arthritis, especially if you're experiencing a flare-up.

12. **Consider attending a local arthritis support group**, no matter what your age. Support group members understand your struggles because they face or have faced the same challenges. To find an arthritis support group in your community, see the Resources section at the end of this chapter or consult the Yellow Pages of your telephone book.

    The Arthritis Foundation's Discussion Boards[1] offer online forums for communicating with others. There are forums for research, just- diagnosed, young adults, advocacy, coping, parenting, and more. Use these boards to connect with others who live with arthritis, to make new friends, and to create a circle of support for yourself. You might also consider starting a small group that gets together for lunch or coffee. Being with others who have your illness can alleviate fears rather than worsen them.

Understanding and Managing Arthritis and Related Conditions

Your Unique Needs

13. **Recognize your uniqueness.** Everyone is different; you have your own unique symptoms and responses to everything, from activity to medications. Be aware of what works and what doesn't seem to work for you.

14. **Work with your doctor to find what works for you.** If one medication is not helping, ask to try another. If side effects are worse than the original condition, speak up. Be an active participant in your healthcare.

15. **Ask to see an occupational or physical therapist** who can assess your limitations and help you work with your body to achieve less pain and stiffness.

16. **Find a way to include gentle exercise in your daily routine.** Gentle exercise helps to relieve pain, keep stiffness at bay, and improve your overall well-being. Even a few minutes of gentle stretching each day can make a world of difference in how you feel now and in the progression of your disease. Ask your doctor about a referral to an exercise physiologist who can help you design a gentle routine based on your specific needs. See if your clinic offers tai chi or yoga classes, or join a health club with a warm-water pool that allows you to swim or do water aerobics with less strain on your body (the water helps to support you).

Staying Positive

Attitude

17. **Keep balance in your life.** Prioritize, eliminate, consolidate, and streamline activities in all aspects of your life.

18. **Take care of yourself.** Make compromises. Do the things that are important to you and your family and try to eliminate unnecessary or difficult tasks. Be selfish with how you spend your time and energy. Give yourself permission to rest. Put your feet up when possible, and take the word "should" out of your vocabulary.

19. **Pace your activities and rest before you're exhausted.** Try to break any given activity into a series of smaller tasks. If need be, enlist the help of others.

20. **Eat a healthy diet.** Don't skip meals or resort to junk food. Our bodies need regular meals and whole foods—filled with essential vitamins, minerals, and proteins—to build and grow. This is especially important when you have an illness. Ask your doctor whether an anti-inflammatory diet would be helpful.

21. **Ask for help when you need it.** Don't look at it as giving in; see asking for help as making an intelligent decision that will make your life easier, healthier, and safer. And remember—when you ask someone to help you, you are giving them the opportunity to do a good deed for someone else. So, do something nice for someone else—ask for their help.

Support

22. **Learn about your medical condition** along with current research and treatments that will help you keep a positive attitude and give you hope for the future. Go to the library, search reputable sites on the Internet, or

contact research organizations such as the Arthritis Foundation, American College of Rheumatology,[2] the National Institute of Arthritis and Musculoskeletal and Skin Diseases (NIAMS),[3] the National Institutes of Health (NIH)[4] health information pages, or general medical sites such as Web MD[5] or the NIH-sponsored MedLine Plus.[6] These support services, and more, are listed at the end of the chapter.

23. **Ask your doctor about support groups in your area.** If you have been diagnosed with a chronic illness or disease, it is good to know you are not alone. Local support groups provide understanding, encouragement, and information about treatments and resources available for you and your family in your home area. Often hospitals, HMOs, and clinics offer "coping-type" support groups for people with chronic illness or those going through life-altering changes. If going to a support group scares you, see if you can attend over the phone or talk to one or more of the members one-on-one. In knowledge and understanding is power to relieve your fears and live a better, more active life.

24. **Consider a service dog for help and companionship.** If your arthritic condition severely hampers your mobility, a trained service dog may be helpful to you[7-8]. In addition to providing companionship, these dogs may be trained to respond to about 90 commands to help with day-to-day activities such as retrieving dropped items or items from shelves, opening doors, carrying items, pulling wheelchairs up ramps, turning on lights, and assisting with counter exchanges at banks and stores—tasks that can assist both children and adults in achieving greater safety and independence. Many organizations rescue dogs from animal shelters, providing yet another valuable service to the community. When choosing a service dog, be sure that

adequate attention is given to matching your needs and desires with the dog's abilities and personality.

Community Resources

25. Your local library is a wealth of information and resources. The reference desk librarians can answer almost any question, from what is the capitol of Zambia to the address and phone number of a local restaurant. They are a wonderful resource in locating contact information for support groups and organizations and helping you with Internet searches. You can reserve books over the phone or online, and the library will notify you when they are available; some communities even have volunteers who will drop off and pick up your library books at no charge. Find more tips on how to utilize library services in Chapter 7.

26. Contact your local independent living center. Every state has independent living centers (ILCs) whose mission is to help the elderly and people with disabilities continue to live independently. Most centers have adaptive gadgets and devices you can borrow at no cost for a trial period. ILCs also have a vast computer database of those companies and manufacturers that make these products. Your city or county human services office or arthritis support agency should be able to assist you in finding the ILC nearest you.[9]

27. Apply for disabled parking privileges. If you have difficulty walking, you may qualify for a disabled parking permit. With the permit, you can park in specially designated stalls closer to the entrance of doctor's offices, stores, and businesses. You may also be able to park in regular stalls near where you are going without paying for parking. Along with your application, you will need a signed statement from your physician verifying your need for a temporary or permanent permit.

Ask your state Department of Transportation about qualifications and how to apply.

Living and Working Smart

Energy-saving Techniques

New technology is created everyday that may make it easier for you to do what you want to do. Invest in devices that will conserve energy and reduce stress and strain on affected joints.

28. **Use labor-saving devices.** Electric or power-assisted can and jar openers, power blinds, robotic vacuums, front-loading washers, self-timing ovens, and slow cookers—use any device, large or small, that will make your life easier.

29. **Let technology aid you.** Remote controlled TVs and entertainment systems, cordless phones, and other devices save steps. Speakerphones, answering machines, and wireless intercoms can be used to save time and energy. Computers are good for keeping records, keeping a journal, and writing letters. An electronic Personal Data Assistant (PDA) can help you keep track of appointments and your schedule. An Internet connection can expand your research capabilities and provide opportunities to communicate with others who have a similar condition. Keep abreast of new technology and make full use of every option helpful to you.

30. **Arrange your home for your convenience.** Arrange furniture, lighting, and frequently used items in ways that help rather than hinder you. Sometimes this means placing furniture in strategic locations to help you walk from room to room or putting a chair halfway down a long hallway so you can rest. Or, it can mean duplicating items such as cleaning supplies—one set for each

floor of your home—and storing the items near where they are used most frequently.

31. **Keep things that you use frequently readily accessible.** Avoid the frequency of opening the flatware drawer by placing the caddy on the countertop or, for a more decorative appearance, stand knives, forks, and spoons in pretty containers. Place oversized cooking utensils in a pretty crock near the stove. Roll kitchen towels and dishcloths and place in a basket near the sink. Do the same with bathroom towels and place them within easy reach of where you need them. Find alternative ways to store everyday items within easy reach.

Plan and Use Time Wisely

Prioritize

32. **Concentrate on the important things.** Conserve your energy for the things that are most important to you, and delegate or even forget the rest. Spending quality time with your family is more important than having a perfectly clean house or manicured lawn. Choose clothing that does not need ironing; get an easy care haircut; and use pre-cut, washed, or prepared items to shortcut meal preparation. Make choices to enhance your life and well-being instead of worrying about the details.

33. **Prioritize chores into categories** like "must be done," "should be done," and "nice to get done." Begin each day by tackling the "must be done" items, taking short breaks between them if necessary. Less important tasks and jobs can be assigned to family members or moved to another day.

34. **Use online, telephone, mail-order, and delivery services as much as possible.** You can shop when it is con-

venient for you and not worry about running out of energy.

Lists and Reminders

35. **Keep a "to do" list.** It feels good to realize how much you accomplish each day. And, for those times when you can't seem to get anything done, look at all the things on your list that you have completed.

36. **Carry a small spiral bound notebook with you.** Jot down information you need to remember and things you need to get done. If you attach one end of a piece of string or ribbon to a pen or pencil and the other end to the spiral binding, you'll always have a writing utensil handy.

37. **Use self-sticking notes.** Self-adhesive note pads stay in place and won't slide around when you write lists for errands, make grocery lists, or take telephone messages. Put sticky notes on the door, so that you remember to take necessary items with you when leaving home, put them on a family members' mirror to remind them of important engagements or errands, or use them to mark your place in a book or remind you where to start when you come back to a project.

38. **Use large chalkboards or dry-erase boards** to keep track of appointments and tasks. Board entries are easy to update or erase, and you don't have to worry about writing in small spaces or losing your notes. You may want to use different colors to code the messages for family members so everyone will know at a glance which pertain to them.

39. **Manage your appointments and to-do lists electronically.** If it is easier to type than hold a pen and write, keep important information and your calendar on a computer or PDA. Shop around for a PDA that is

lightweight, with buttons that are easy for you to reach and push.

Staying Organized

40. **Create a calendar for sending greeting cards.** At the beginning of each year, start with a new calendar that has a square for each day, and write the names of people celebrating birthdays, holidays, graduations, wedding anniversaries, whatever, in the appropriate square. Purchase cards for each person, sort them according to the month in which they must be mailed, and file in an easy-to-access accordion file so they are ready to send when those special days come up. (You might also designate a file slot for sympathy, get well, new baby, and "just because" cards.) If you prefer, keep your calendar on your computer and set it to remind you to send cards on the appropriate days. Software programs such as American Greetings CreataCard or Art Explosion Greeting Card Factory Deluxe allow you to print custom cards at home. Find software at your office supply store or at Amazon.com.

41. **Use zipper-type storage bags to store important papers.** Gallon bags are big enough for most papers to slide in and out easily—just label and keep in a box or drawer. Some zipper-type bags are easier to use than others; experiment with different brands and styles.

42. **Use your home computer to keep paperwork organized** and help family members who must assist with your personal business. Create a document entitled WHEREITIS and list the location of important or valuable papers. For security purposes, protect the document with a password that you give only to those who might need to access the file. Keep a back-up of the file on an external storage device (CD, flash drive, etc.) in a

separate location, like a safe deposit box or at the home
of a family member. If you don't have a computer, write
or type a master list and keep a copy in a safe location
away from home.

43. **Hang a multipocket shoe bag inside a closet or behind
any door to help organize your bills.** Label each
pocket—health insurance, car insurance, car payments,
utility bills, mortgage, charitable contributions, clubs/
organizations, newspaper/magazine subscriptions,
etc.—and use small sticky notes or a grease pencil to
indicate due dates. You'll know at a glance which bills
need to be paid and when.

44. **Keep small cleaning or craft supplies in a storage bin**
with a handle so you can carry the bin with you as
needed. If possible, purchase a ruler, stapler, scissors, and
tape for each family member who is old enough to use
them safely. Put the owner's name on each item, so that
everyone has their own supply. Family members will no
longer borrow (and forget to return) your supplies.

RESOURCES

Support Organizations

1. **Arthritis Foundation**
   P.O. Box 7669
   Atlanta, GA 30357-0669
   800-283-7800
   www.arthritis.org

2. **American College of Rheumatology**
   1800 Century Place, Suite 250
   Atlanta, GA 30345-4300
   404-633-3777
   www.rheumatology.org

3. **National Institute of Arthritis and Musculoskeletal and Skin Diseases (NIAMS)**
National Institutes of Health
1 AMS Circle
Bethesda, MD 20892-3675
301-495-4484
Toll Free: 877-22-NIAMS (226-4267)
TTY: 301–565–2966
www.niams.nih.gov

4. **National Institutes for Health (NIH)**
9000 Rockville Pike
Bethesda, Maryland 20892
301-496-4000
www.health.nih.gov

5. **Web MD**
www.WebMD.com

6. **MedLine Plus**
www.MedlinePlus.gov

Service Dogs

7. **Assistance Dog United Campaign**
1221 Sebastopol Road
Santa Rosa, CA 95407
800-284-DOGS (3647)
www.AssistanceDogUnitedCampaign.org

8. **Sterling Service Dogs**
3715 E. Fifteen Mile Road
Sterling Heights, MI 48310
586-977-9716
www.SterlingServiceDogs.org.

This organization may be able to custom train a dog for an owner's specific needs. Also check out the Service-dogs Internet listserv by sending a message with a blank subject line to majordomo@acpub.duke.edu with the following words in the body of the message: subscribe service-dogs. You can send messages to the list at service-dogs@acpub.duke.edu.

Independent Living

9. Independent Living Centers
www.ilusa.com

CHAPTER 2

Empowering Yourself

Having arthritis can sometimes feel like you're in an unstable canoe with jet skiers unexpectedly whizzing by, threatening to tip you over. Some days you can tackle the world; other days, you can hardly get out of bed. It's difficult to stay positive when there's no way to predict good times and bad. A lot of energy is wasted on feelings of anger, helplessness, frustration, and guilt—energy that could be used more productively. To channel your energy in positive, pleasant, and productive ways, here are more ideas to help you maximize the good days and minimize the bad.

45. **Accept that you'll have good days and bad.** When things are more difficult, choose activities that require less energy and stamina. Put pictures in the photo album, pay bills, read, make out the grocery list, or use the phone to talk to a friend, make appointments, or track down merchandise. At the end of the day, you'll feel good knowing that you didn't "waste" the day. And, if all you can do is sleep and watch a movie, know that you did the best thing for that day and took care of you.

46. **Be honest with yourself and others.** People are able to accept you and what you can offer if you are open and honest with them. Explain why you may not be able to coach your son's soccer team this year, then offer to do a job that requires less active participation. Remember, you are not alone; many people have limited their commitments for a variety of reasons.

47. **Tell people how they can help.** If you want to be dropped off at the door instead of walking the extra distance from the parking lot, tell your friend. If a full glass of water is too heavy to lift, ask to have it filled only half way, and tell them why. If at times, it's too difficult to go out, and you don't want to be alone, ask a friend to come over. It's your responsibility to tell people specifically how they can help you.

48. **Find new ways to do the things you like to do.** Don't stop doing things you enjoy, such as traveling, gardening, painting, crafts, and the like just because it takes a little more planning and preparation. Modify your activities. Use adapted devices. Stay involved.

49. **Plan things to look forward to.** Set small short-term goals for yourself. Invite friends over to play cards or watch a football game. Plan to see a new movie in town or attend a family reunion or an upcoming birthday party. Then, even if a bad day sneaks in, you'll have something to look forward to.

50. **Anticipate problems and their solutions.** Whenever you plan an activity, discuss potential problems and make contingency plans to provide alternatives if problems arise. Rehearse what you would do if ... the car broke down on the highway, you missed your plane connection, or you couldn't find an accessible bathroom. Taking risks can be stressful, but careful planning and preparation will reduce stress and make activities more enjoyable.

51. **Look for the positive aspects of what's happening to you.** Do you have more time for family and friends? Are you more organized? Are your children more independent than other children their age? Are you finding new abilities and talents you never knew you had?

52. **Concentrate on your abilities.** Even if your body is betraying you, use your mind to overcome obstacles. Remember, you haven't changed, just your ability to do things has changed. Face one day at a time and feel good about yourself and how resourceful you can be.

Whether you've had arthritis for years, or you've just been diagnosed, here are ideas for being proactive:

Protecting Joints

53. **Work with a physical or occupational therapist** to find ways to eliminate undue stress on affected body parts. Ask your doctor for a recommendation and/or referral.

54. **Concentrate on using larger muscle groups.** Whenever possible, use your arms, shoulders, legs, and back to reduce wear and tear on your hands, knees, and other more arthritis-susceptible joints.

55. **Avoid bending over repeatedly when you work.** Keep a small waste basket in your workspace and, as you work, throw in items to be discarded or recycled. Carry the basket with you until your job is finished. Then throw away or recycle all the unwanted items at once.

56. **Walk as you vacuum.** Standing still while pushing and pulling the vacuum puts more stress on your back.

57. **Carry items in a backpack,** instead of a shoulder-slung purse or bag, to help you keep your balance while walking. AmeriBag makes a stylish, ergonomically designed bag that hugs your body and distributes the weight of the bag across your hips and back.[1] The tendency is to overfill bags, so keep your bag or backpack small and carry only what you really need.

58. **Use an Armrest Organizer instead of a purse.** If grasping the handles of a purse is uncomfortable, the

Armrest Organizer,[2] designed to slip over the arm of a wheelchair or walker, can be carried on your arm instead of in your hands or over your shoulder. Adjust the Velcro fasteners to fit, and the flip top pouch rests flush against your body, wheelchair, or scooter, offering quick access yet secure storage. Check out the Resources section at the end of the chapter for more information.

Managing Pain

59. **Wear driving gloves for hand pain.** If your hands and fingers are very sensitive and painful, driving gloves (the leather type that covers your hand and leaves the tips of your fingers free) might give you enough support and protection to make daily activities less painful. Try them when carrying packages or groceries, carrying hangers, changing bedding—anytime your hands give you trouble. Elastic gloves, designed for carpal tunnel or computer use, are another option. Ask your healthcare professional about the type of gloves you should wear and where to find them.

60. **Put your feet up.** To take pressure off your legs and back when seated in a chair, car, or bench, do not let your legs dangle. If you do not have a footstool, put a box or books under your feet.

61. **Stay warm.** Cold joints are often stiff and sore joints. Here are some ways to keep your body warm and more limber:
    - *Fleece or electric mattress pads* provide additional warmth underneath you to help you sleep better and wake with less pain. Kerry Hills Farm[3] is the maker of Surround Ewe™ Sleep Systems, 100 percent organic underquilts, comforters, and pillows filled with wool batting, which has a natural resilience and springiness for even weight distribution. Wool also has

natural insulation properties that work with your body to regulate your temperature, warming you quickly in the winter and wicking away moisture to cool you in the summer.

- *Try down-filled comforters* for lightweight warmth. Down-filled comforters often provide greater warmth and are lighter than polyester or quilted bedding. Dress up comforters with a duvet cover to match your décor.
- *Try sleeping with an electric blanket or mattress pad,* if morning stiffness and pain makes it difficult for you to get out of bed. The heat of the blanket throughout the night helps to keep muscles and joints more flexible. If your electric blanket powers down or off overnight, try turning up the heat for 20 minutes before getting up.
- *Take a hot shower to start your day.* Slowly stretch and move under the water to reduce stiffness. If dry skin is then a problem, slather on warm olive oil (set an unbreakable container inside your shower to warm) or a highly emollient lotion afterward.
- *Wear wrist warmers.* Wear long gloves, with the fingers cut out, or sew a fleece sleeve that covers your wrist and the palm of your hand (cut a hole for your thumb about an inch from the top), leaving your fingers free to type, sew, read, write, or work. Wear them in the house or don them before putting on your coat or jacket to keep out cold drafts. You might also purchase Wristies®,[4] which come in a variety of sizes and colors, both heated and unheated versions, and also in a longer version called Sleeves that covers over your elbow.
- *Keep your feet warm.* Your big toe is your body's thermostat, so keep it warm and your whole body will be warm. Wear wool socks, fleece slippers, and/or leg warmers to stay warm when you are sitting or lying down. Happy Toes,[5] soft polyester fleece slippers

with a removable, microwavable pouch filled with rice, buckwheat hulls, and a hint of cloves, lavender, and chamomile, provide instant heat to cold feet and soothing relief for aching and sore muscles.

- *Make your own heat pack.* Place 2 cups of rice or buckwheat hulls (available at a natural foods store) in a sock, tie the end, microwave for 2 minutes, and place wherever soothing heat is desired. For larger areas, place more rice or buckwheat in a small pillow case.

- *Carry hand and foot warmers with you for instant warming* when you need it. Hand and foot warmers that skiers, hunters, and other winter outdoor enthusiasts use are an inexpensive way to stay warm for several hours. Slip one in your pocket when going out in the cold for a quick warm-up anytime. Or, place foot warmers (which do not get as hot as hand warmers) on the top of your hand inside a mitten or glove, and they will warm your fingers and circulate the warmth up your arm. If your feet get cold, a foot warmer placed against your upper thigh will warm the blood headed for your toes; hold in place by slipping under long underwear, leggings, or tights. You can find hand and foot warmers at ski shops, outdoor outfitters, and in the sporting goods section of large discount stores.

62. **Use a hand massager or vibrating head and neck pillow** to help ease the pain when you are bothered by stiff, tight, or achy muscles. Some vibrators or massagers are designed to hold in your hand and massage the spine; others cover the back and/or seat of your chair for an all-over massage experience. Some just vibrate; others have rolling parts inside that massage more vigorously. Some allow the addition of soothing heat with your massage. There's even a neck pillow designed to strap onto the back of an office chair or car seat. Remove the detachable strap, and you can position the pillow to massage your neck, back, shoulders,

legs, and feet. Because the pillow vibrates quietly, you won't disturb others if you use it in bed or during a meeting, and it is great for long car rides. Vibrating massagers are sold in drug and department stores.

Conserving Energy

63. **Sit down while you work.** If you have pain in your legs, knees, or feet, take the strain of gravity off by sitting down to work. Even tall counters, such as those in the kitchen and work room, can be made easier to work at using tall stools—some even come with rollers to make getting around easier.

64. **Combine errands as much as possible.** If you are making the effort to get dressed and get in the car, don't just go out for one thing—conserve gas and energy by making a list and running all your errands at one time. Be efficient—list your errands in the order you wish to run them, making a circle from home to the farthest point and home again or, if you might run out of time or energy, prioritize by importance and do the most important things first.

65. **Spread out high-energy tasks.** Instead of trying to do the laundry, get groceries, and clean the house all in one day, spread these activities out throughout the week. Give yourself time to rest, perhaps even a rest day, in between high-intensity activities.

Coping with Change

66. **Adapt to changes.** Receiving a diagnosis can be distressing, and adjusting to the effects of the disease can be challenging, but you can still lead a remarkably unlimited life if you put your mind to it. By adapting your routine, making your home more accessible, and keeping a positive outlook, you have the power to take control of your life and rise above the challenges you face.

67. **Go with the flow.** The course of arthritis is unpredictable, and it can affect your life in many ways. It can be as simple as morning stiffness that dissipates with a hot shower, or it can be a painful and disabling condition that restricts your ability to do simple, everyday activities. Some days it's easy to cope with the challenges; other days, it would be easier to give up and throw in the towel. There is no doubt about it—living with a chronic illness is difficult, but allow yourself to go with the flow of your illness. Getting angry or upset only makes matters worse.

68. **Make the most of your life.** Living with a chronic illness like arthritis often takes people on a journey they never planned on. Simple tasks like buttoning a shirt, opening a jar, or climbing stairs require more thought and planning, and "normal" activities, like walking, exercising, driving, and working present daily reminders of how life has changed. Admit your limitations, and then find a way to work around them. The sooner you can accept whatever changes come your way and find a way to live with them instead of fight against them, the happier and healthier you will be.

Staying Mobile

Reachers

69. **Reachers** allow you to pick up things off the floor without bending or to reach items on higher shelves while seated. They come in various lengths, weights, and means of operation.
    - *Trigger grip reachers* have a hand grip shaped similar to a pistol that can be operated by squeezing your finger.
    - *Full-grasp handgrip reachers* allow you to squeeze with all your fingers.

- *A locking mechanism reacher* enables you to hold an object tightly without continuing to grasp the handle tightly.
- *Sticky pads or magnets* at the ends of some reachers help with picking up lightweight or metal objects.
- *Rubber grippers or vinyl-covered tips* give better holding power.
- *Battery-operated reachers* automatically open and close gripping jaws with a light push on a rocker switch.
- *Folding reachers* fold in half for traveling or storage, and some come with carrying attachments that clamp the reacher to walkers and wheelchairs.

Your local arthritis chapter or human services agency may help you to locate a resource (independent living center, support group, home health agency, or drug store) that can help you find the style that would be most helpful for you.

Canes, Walking Sticks, and Walkers

70. **Use a cane or walking stick** to reduce pressure on the hip joint by 20–30 percent and result in less pain and fatigue. Proper cane height and usage is important. The top of the cane's handle should reach your wrist when you are standing with arms at your side. Hold the cane or stick on the unaffected side of your body, for best support. Choose from a variety of materials and styles, including one with a four-foot base (a quad cane) that stands on its own.

71. **Carry a collapsible stool cane.** A cane that opens into a seat is a handy thing when you go to museums and art galleries, for hobbies like bird watching, and for waiting in lengthy lines and check outs. Look for these in drug or medical supply stores or online cane stores.[6]

72. **Purchase an adjustable walking staff** and use it when you need a little extra balance or support. Designed for hikers and walkers, several types of lightweight, collapsible, and durable walking poles are available that easily adjust to the correct length yet pack easily into a suitcase when traveling. Purchase at outdoor recreation stores.

73. **Cover your cane handle for better grip.** If you use a cane and find it too cold or slippery to grasp while wearing mittens or gloves, sew, knit, or crochet a small sleeve to fit snugly over the handle. The knit glove and knit cover will cling together and keep the handle from slipping. You can accomplish the same result by wrapping fleece or rubber waffle material over the top of the cane and securing it with rubber bands or by using a section of leather steering wheel cover, available in the automotive section of discount stores.

74. **Choose a walker that is right for you.** If you need more support than a cane or walking stick can give, consider a walker. Walkers today are not as clunky or hard to use as they once were. Some sleek styles come with wheels, handbrakes, a basket for your stuff, and even a place to sit and rest. As a bonus, you can use the walker as a rolling seat or to transport things in the kitchen, laundry—almost anywhere.

75. **Use baby shoes to keep your walker from running away.** If your walker runs away from you, most people slow it down by cutting a slot in a tennis ball and putting one on each leg. For a cute alternative, use baby shoes instead of tennis balls—you'll be the talk of the town.

76. **Use nylon glides to reduce friction on carpet.** If you use a walker primarily on carpeted surfaces, add nylon glides to keep from catching on the nap. Choose from a variety of styles. Star Glides™ self-align with the floor, allowing you to lift and place your walker with less

effort and more stability. Simply replace the rubber tips on the bottom of the back legs with the glides. Look for these and other walker accessories at drug or home health stores.[7]

RESOURCES

Ergonomic Bags

1. **AmeriBag Inc.**
   Consumer Services Department
   5 AmeriBag Drive
   Kingston, NY 12401
   888-758-1636
   www.AmeriBag.com

2. **Armrest Organizer**
   CaseLogic
   6303 Dry Creek Parkway
   Longmont, CO 80503
   888-666-5780
   www.CaseLogic.com

Warm-ups

3. **Wool Underquilts**
   Surround Ewe™ Sleep Systems
   N1237 Franklin Road
   Oconomowoc, WI 53066
   888-WOOLBED (966-5233)
   www.KerryHillsFarm.com

4. **Wristies**
   Wannalancit Mills
   650 Suffolk Street, Suite G-5
   Lowell, MA 01854
   800-811-8290
   www.wristies.com

5. **Happy Toes**
   The Happy Company
   26203 Production Avenue, Suite 4
   Hayward, CA 94545
   800-486-2896
   www.TheHappyCompany.com

Canes and Walkers

6. **www.canemart.com**
   www.FashionableCanes.com
   www.TheWalkingCaneStore.com
   www.WalkingCaneDepot.com

7. **Walker Accessories**
   The Wright Stuff, Inc.
   135 Floyd G. Harrell Drive
   Grenada, MS 38901
   877-750-0376
   www.Mobility-Aids.com

CHAPTER 3

Managing Medical Issues

The day I was diagnosed with my chronic illness, I entered a whole new world—a world that now included doctors, nurses, pharmacists, and therapists. And then there were all the appointments, medical terms, procedures, tests, and medications. I learned early on that you need to stay organized and take an active role in managing your healthcare; doing so gives you some control over your illness and assures family and friends that you are coping well with your new reality.

77. **Stick with one practice group to keep medical care simple.** When your doctors and specialists belong to the same medical practice or health maintenance organization (HMO), all your medical records are in one place and managing your medical care is easier. In addition, seeing other specialists in the group (orthopedists, physiatrists, occupational/physical therapists, speech/language pathologists, and psychologists/psychiatrists) can reduce the hassles of obtaining referrals and filling out endless paperwork at new doctors' offices. Be sure to find out if your insurance covers home health services for medical management in the home, physical therapy visits, and so on—you may be surprised by what is covered.

78. **Choose doctors whom you like and with whom you have a good rapport.** A healthcare provider's bedside manner is extremely important. Research shows that patients who are satisfied with their physicians are healthier overall than those who are not. If a friend or acquaintance recommends a doctor, keep in mind that you may have different experiences, opinions, or preferences. If your doctor doesn't treat you with respect, listen to you, or see you as a whole person—as an individual, a family member, a person with a career and a social life—find one who does. Obtain a copy of the Patient's Bill of Rights and make sure your healthcare providers adhere to it. It is important that you stick up for yourself, be your own advocate, and take responsibility for your medical care.

79. **Keep a copy of your medical records.** Most states have enacted laws that give patients access to their hospital and physicians' records. Access to records may be more difficult in states where such legislation does not exist, but no state specifically denies access to your records. Whether you move often, travel frequently, see doctors in other cities, or just like to keep your own medical records up-to-date, ask for copies of your files at the completion of each appointment. Because of the Health Insurance Portability and Accountability Act (HIPAA), doctors, hospitals, and clinics are only allowed to give medical papers/reports to the patient in person. There may be a cost to obtain your medical records and you will have to sign a release form.

80. **Be proactive—learn more about your illness.** Another way to get involved in your own medical care is to learn more about it. The Arthritis Foundation provides accurate, up-to-date information about treatments, research, and support services. Enlist your friends and family members to do research, too; it will give you all something positive to do. Collect infor-

mation from newspapers, magazines, and medical journals. If there is a university near your home, visit the medical school library or search for reputable resources on the Internet. Share information and learn together. Bring articles and information to your next doctor's appointment, so that you can discuss the findings and see how they relate to your case. You may even find that you've read medical journal articles before your doctor has had a chance to read them. It's important to be proactive when it comes to your health, and most doctors like working with well-informed patients.

Here are more tips, strategies, and ideas to help you manage your medical care.

Record Keeping and Research

81. **Keep a medical history.** Prepare a chronological list of medical treatments, surgeries, hospitalizations, and medications. The list comes in handy when answering physicians' and pharmacists' questions. You can create your own in a binder or purchase Your Personal Health and Medical History[1]—an organizer divided into ten categories (personal information, medications, hospitalizations, emergency contacts, etc.) and filled with detailed forms that are easy to fill out. The organizer also contains 18 legal documents, including Power of Attorney, healthcare directives, and the like that you can fill out as you need. A medical history binder is an invaluable resource for keeping all your medical records centralized—especially in case of emergency. If you prefer, you can get a software version to use on your computer.

82. **Copy your medical history onto a computer flash drive.** Once you enter your medical information onto your computer, including personal information, insurance

and physician information, medications and allergies, medical history, special needs, even a living will and healthcare durable power of attorney, make a copy on a portable USB flash drive. Easier to update than a CD file, these small "memory sticks" will clip onto a key chain or slip easily into a pocket or purse, allowing you to transfer medical information quickly and easily when you meet with new doctors or end up in the emergency room when traveling. These drives can be plugged into any computer USB port, making all the data instantly available to doctors and hospitals anywhere you go. For added security, you might want to make two paper copies of important reports and keep the second at a relative's house. Be sure to keep this information up to date.

83. **Consult a source for drug information in lay language.** Drug reactions can be fatal. Before taking a new medication, educate yourself. Ask your pharmacist for written instructions, common uses for the drug, and a list of side effects, then compare them to the information your doctor gave you. If the doctor's instructions do not match with what the pharmacist says, consult the *USP DI, Volume II, Advice for the Patient: Drug Information in Lay Language* at your local library (or call the reference librarian at your local library to help you). If you note discrepancies or have questions, contact your doctor for an explanation.

84. **Use reputable online medical sources.** Researching your condition online can be valuable but stick to reputable sources like the Arthritis Foundation, The Centers for Disease Control, and other government-sponsored sites. See the Resources section of Chapter 1 for more sources of reputable online information.

Doctors and Appointments

Scheduling Appointments

85. **Schedule an appointment at a time of day when your doctor is less busy and/or at an optimal time for your energy level.** When you have arthritis, you may want to request the first appointment after lunch. Although emergencies happen to alter your doctor's schedule, it is less likely that she will be backed up at this time, and you will get in and out more quickly.

86. **Ask to be put on the cancellation list.** If the doctor has no openings, and you feel you need to see your doctor soon, ask the receptionist if there is a list of patients who might be able to come in on short notice in the event of a cancellation; if so, ask to be put on the list. If you have not heard from the receptionist within a few days, call back and ask about any cancellations.

87. **Make appointments with new specialists through your doctor.** When the appointment request comes from another doctor, you will often get in to see the specialist sooner.

88. **Give yourself enough lead time for appointments.** If you are seeing a specialist with whom it takes weeks or months to schedule an appointment, put a reminder in your calendar to call and schedule an appointment two or three months before you need to see your doctor again.

89. **Discuss how much time you will have to spend with the doctor** when you make your appointment. Depending on the reason for your doctor's visit, you may be scheduled for as little as five minutes or as much as half an hour. If you feel you will need more time, ask for it.

90. **Let the doctor's office know that you use special hand-icapped transportation** to medical or dental appointments. Most people don't realize that special transportation often must be scheduled 24 hours in advance, and you must include not only when you need to be delivered but also when you need to be picked up from your appointment. Let the scheduler know how important having an on-time appointment is, and ask them to call you as soon as they are aware that the doctor (or dentist) is running late so that you can try to adjust your transportation arrangements.

91. **Schedule the next appointment before you leave the doctor's office.** If you need to schedule appointments on a regular basis (such as monthly monitoring), make your next appointment before you leave the doctor's office. It may be helpful to schedule frequent appointments, such as weekly treatments up to four weeks in advance.

92. **Schedule annual appointments around annual events such as birthdays, anniversaries, or the start of the year.** This not only helps you to remember your appointment, it may also give you an opportunity to schedule at a time that is less busy for both you and your doctor.

93. **Bring a friend or family member along on your appointment.** Between the two of you, you will remember more of what the doctor has to say about your condition and treatment options. Take notes or tape-record your visit so that you can review your doctor's explanations and answers to your questions after you get home.

In the days prior to your appointment:

94. **Plan ahead for your appointment.** If you find the fast pace of medical appointments disconcerting, and you

routinely come away with questions you forgot to ask your doctor, a little advance planning might help. Think through the things you want to discuss with your doctor and write them down in order of importance.

95. **Consider keeping a diary of your symptoms**, of your ups and downs, good times and bad, so the doctor can gain a better understanding of how you're doing, especially when new medications are introduced. You may also want a family member or friend to keep a similar diary, recording their perceptions; having more than one perspective can often give the physician a clearer picture of how well a treatment or medication is working.

96. **Ask the nurse about any tests or procedures that might be performed at the visit.** If these are upsetting, let the doctor know, so that you can work together to prepare yourself and alleviate any fears or unnecessary discomfort.

The day of your appointment:

97. **Call the doctor's office to see if the doctor is running on schedule.** If you know a delay may be possible, you might choose to alter when you arrive, take a snack, or bring a book with you. Confirm the appointment time and what time you need to leave home.

98. **Take a favorite stuffed animal, some small toys, or a favorite book** to entertain your child while waiting. Leave other children at home, or bring another adult along to watch them.

The following checklist will help you prepare for your next appointment:

99. **Write down things you want to tell the doctor** including a review of all medicines, vitamins, hormones, or

steroids you may be taking and any changes in your weight, sleep, temper, stress levels, or menstrual cycle.

100. **Make a list of questions to ask the doctor.** What are your concerns about your health? Do you have any specific worries? Should any screening tests be considered? Are you up to date on all routine exams and vaccinations?

101. **Make sure your medical history is current.** Inform your doctor of any family history of arthritis, heart disease, stroke, Alzheimer's, cancer, or other diseases.

102. **Know what procedures the doctor plans to carry out.** Review what preparations you need to make ahead of time (no food or water after midnight, etc.) and follow instructions carefully.

103. **Take along a pen and paper to make notes** of what your doctor says. Always ask your doctor to explain anything about your treatment program that you don't understand. Try repeating back what you think you heard, and ask your doctor for written information about your condition.

104. **Take along plain self-adhesive stick-on labels.** If your doctor prescribes a medication, note what the doctor tells you and, when you get the prescription filled, stick it on the bottle for future reference.

Medications

105. **Use your pharmacist as a resource.** Because they work with medications every day, pharmacists are often very knowledgeable about how certain drugs might affect your body, their side effects, and any possible contraindications or undesirable interactions that could occur between new drugs prescribed and those you are already taking. Use one pharmacy, so that you have a complete record of your medications, including drugs prescribed by multiple doctors.

Be sure you and your family know how any pre-scribed medications work, what the side effects are, and any symptoms you should report to your doctor. Do not take any medication, including nonprescription products such as vitamins, dietary supplements, allergy and cold medicines, pain relievers, or herbal remedies, without first consulting your doctor.

106. **Ask your doctor if generic drugs may be used to fill your prescription.** Generics are less expensive than brand-name drugs. Ask if the generic drug differs from the brand-name drug in terms of efficacy. Also, ask your doctor for booklets or other literature on the use and possible side effects of prescribed medications.

107. **Discuss timing of medications with your doctor.** Med-ications can have different effects on different people. Timing your medication to your personal body clock can maximize benefits. If your medication affects your energy, mood, or wears off at an inopportune time, dis-cuss with your physician the possibility of taking it on a different schedule. If an early morning increase in symptoms is trying, ask about taking long-acting tablets at bedtime to help you wake up more comfortably.

108. **Try medications in longer-acting or time-release ver-sions.** If you do not have to take medication as often, there are fewer pill bottles to open, pills to take, and less stress about missing a dose. Ask your doctor if a long-acting or time-release version is appropriate for you.

109. **Create a daily medicine routine.** Create a written schedule, with space for each medication and when to take it (time of day, before, during, or after meals), and keep it in a handy location where you can check off each dose as you take it. Or, purchase plastic daily / weekly pill organizers, available at most pharmacies, so that you will know at a glance if you have taken your meds. If organizing your pills is difficult or stressful,

consider asking your pharmacist to separate your pills into specific doses according to when they should be taken (morning, noon, dinner, bedtime) and to put them into smaller, easy-opening containers.

110. **Keep medications in a decorative tin on a table near a favorite chair or couch.** The tin acts as a reminder to take the meds while eliminating the unsightliness of a bottle-covered table—and it's portable. Of course, if there are children in the house, you will want to keep all medications out of their reach.

111. **Keep extra doses of medication handy.** If possible, keep several doses of medicine in your car, at your workplace, and in your wallet or purse so you will never run out of important medication. Be sure to take this dose and replace it with fresh medication regularly.

RESOURCES

Health and Medical History

1. **Planet Media Group**
   13515 Old Dock Road
   Orlando, FL 32828
   888-669-9697
   www.HealthHistory.com

CHAPTER 4

In Your Home

I spend lots of time in my home, so I've created an environment where I can be safe, productive, and independent. My husband and I made many changes and adaptations to our home ourselves. We installed wireless intercoms to save steps and allow us to communicate between one end of the house and another without shouting; using a lawn chair in the shower made it safer for me to shower while alone in the house; and putting a railing on both sides of the stairway to the basement provided the extra support I needed.

When we built a new home a few years ago, I tried to incorporate additional accessibility features, including:

- **Remote-controlled window shades**—no more stretching or reaching needed
- **Low-height wall thermostats** that make it easier for me to see the temperature and adjust the setting
- **U-shaped handles on the kitchen cabinets** to make them easier to grab and open
- **A comfortable, cushioned lift-chair** for the great room, so I can get in or out of a chair with minimal help, put my feet up, and adjust my position easily
- **A universal remote**[1] programmed to control the lights, TV, DVD player, and fan

In this chapter, you'll find many inexpensive home modifications you can make to improve your safety and comfort without costly remodeling or structural changes. If you find you need more ideas for improving accessibly in your home, ask your doctor to recommend an occupational therapist; she will come to your house to evaluate your surroundings and make suggestions specifically for *you* and *your* living situation.

Should you want or need to make more involved changes to your home that require the help of a professional, ask family members, friends, neighbors, and coworkers for recommendations, or contact your local independent living center (ILC) for the name of a contractor, handyman, or trade professional with expertise in advising people with physical limitations. The ILC belongs to a network of centers across the country that help people with chronic illness and disability with housing, advocacy, transportation, employment, health, and social services issues.

Accessibility and Safety

Safety

112. **Be prepared in case of emergency.** Have a plan of action in case of emergency. Know who you can call if you suddenly need help. Plan escape routes and family meeting locations, program emergency numbers into your phones, and determine contact alternatives such as text messaging or calling an out-of-state relative if local phone service is jammed. Have a ready source of clean drinking water handy and an emergency kit (see next tip for contents). You might even install a back-up generator. Anticipate your needs in a worse-case scenario, and prepare to meet those needs.

113. **Keep an emergency kit ready to grab and go.** In a small, easy-to-reach shoulder bag or backpack, include the following:
     - *Flashlight* with extra batteries
     - *Battery-operated radio* with extra batteries
       (To avoid corrosion, store batteries outside of the device or place a piece of cardboard between the batteries and the battery contacts.)
     - *Extra set of keys* for your house and car

- *Extra pair of glasses*
- *Cash, phone card, or change*, and a duplicate credit card
- *Bottled water* (replace every 6 months)
- *Nonperishable, high-energy food* (dried fruit, nuts, granola bars, peanut butter and crackers)
- *Duplicate driver's license* or identity card and health insurance medical card
- *Copies of your current prescriptions* or a complete list of prescription drugs, with name, dosage, doctor's name, prescription number and pharmacy name, address, and phone number
- *Your list of contacts*, including names and phone numbers of family members, health-care providers, support network members, and key service providers, such as your local emergency management agency, ambulance service, telephone and utility repair, plumber, and building manager or landlord.
- *List of names and model numbers of any medical devices*

Be sure to store your emergency kit in an easily accessible place near the door, so it is easy to grab as you leave the house.

114. **Notify the power company if you use power-dependent equipment.** If you are dependent upon power chairs, electric beds, lifts, and other powered medical devices, obtain a medical form from your power company and have your doctor fill it out, indicating your medical problem and the type of equipment you use. Then, in an emergency, the utility company will make every attempt to restore service to your location as soon as possible. They will also tag your meters so that when repairs, meter changes, or routine maintenance necessitate that the power be cut off, they will notify you ahead of time so you can make back-up arrangements. Keep in mind that if this

equipment is vital, it is your responsibility to have a back-up power source.

115. **Let your local fire department know if you might have difficulty escaping from your home** in the event of a fire. If you have family members living with you, practice a fire drill at home. Show children how the smoke detector works and what it sounds like. Encourage your children to sleep with their doors closed; doing so will buy them time by keeping the smoke and heat out of the room in the event of a fire. Be sure to discuss how important it might be to run to a neighbor's house to get help and call the fire department, emphasizing that leaving the house to get help would not mean they are abandoning their pets or family members. Contact your local fire department for more information on home fire safety.

116. **Plan for a safe exit.** Arrange furniture to allow for easy navigation, especially to exit doors. Create spots for support, using furniture, countertops, grab bars and handles. Add battery-powered emergency lights that go on when the power goes out. Install emergency exit ladders to second-floor bedroom windows. Keep an emergency bag near the door with water, snacks, flashlight, a "space blanket," and copies of important papers, so you can grab it in a hurry when you leave the house.

117. **Keep your address and phone number affixed to each telephone.** If a visitor needs to summon help, he will have this vital information.

118. **Use power strips if electrical wall outlets are difficult to reach or use.** Multiple-outlet power strips are inexpensive enough to use in every room of the house. Plug into any household outlet and place the strips where they are more convenient to reach and use. Most come

with an on/off switch so you can turn everything plugged into the strip (TV, lamp, VCR, etc.) on or off with one switch. The strips are available at most discount and hardware stores.

119. **Use a setback thermostat that allows you to program the furnace and air conditioner.** Program the thermostat once, and it will control the heat, saving you money by automatically lowering the temperature of the house during the night as you sleep or during the day when you're away. In the summer, the thermostat controls the air conditioner in the same way. You can set the temperature to go up a half-hour before you get out of bed to help with morning stiffness and improve your ability to move about. Instead of getting up and down to manipulate little controls to adjust the temperature in your house, the thermostat will do it for you. A variety of setback thermostats are on the market; some allow you to select different settings for weekdays and weekends, while others allow you to program each day individually. Thermostats are generally easy to install and can be purchased from hardware or home-improvement stores. If you want help selecting or installing an automatic thermostat, contact a heating or cooling contractor or electrician in your area.

120. **Install an electronic driveway sensor.**[2] If you need extra time to get to the door to greet visitors, consider installing an electronic driveway sensor that will sound a chime and flash to alert you when a car approaches. For added security, an optional lamp controller will turn on a light or radio. Set it to open a door or gate, or perform different functions based on whether a car is arriving or departing. The remote-controlled device has a 1,000-foot range that will work even in long driveways.

Lighting and Light Switches

121. Replace traditional light switches with rocker-panel switches that require less fine motor control. They can be turned on or off by pressing with an arm, elbow, or palm of the hand. Both lighted and unlighted versions may be found at hardware and home-building supply stores.

122. Control light levels with dimmer switches. So that one person may work or read without disturbing others, install an easy-glide, sliding dimmer switch that will allow you to adjust the light levels in a room. They install easily in place of your regular light switch and can be purchased at most hardware and home-building supply stores.

123. Replace hard-to-reach switches with a switch in the cord. If you have trouble reaching the power switch under the shade of a table lamp, purchase a new lamp with the switch on the power cord or, if you're handy, splice an on/off switch into the cord that plugs into the wall.

124. Install a lamp switch enlarger[3] to make turning lamps on and off easier. This large, three-sided knob slips over or replaces your regular switch.

125. Add a touch-sensitive converter to lamps. Lamps are easier to turn on and off if you install a lamp converter,[4] which fits into the socket and bypasses the on-off switch, making the lamp "touch-sensitive." To install a converter, remove the light bulb and insert the converter into the socket, then replace the light bulb. When you screw in a three-way light bulb, the light gets brighter with each successive touch and then finally turns off. These are available from many lighting and discount department stores.

126. Switch lights on by phone with Light on Call™. Coming home to a dark house can be unsettling. Plug your lamp into Light on Call™,[5] and you can call up to five hours ahead and switch on your lights before you arrive. To give the appearance of someone being home while you are traveling, call home to turn lights on at random times.

Doors, Doorways, and Doorknobs

127. **Replace regular doorknobs with lever handles** or purchase a rubber lever that fits over any standard doorknob. Lever handles are easy to operate—just push down with your hand, arm, or elbow. Purchase these at hardware or building supply stores.

128. **Widen doorways.** If you keep scraping your knuckles when going through a door while using your walker, or wheelchair, widen doorways by one-half to three-quarters of an inch by carefully prying off the door jamb strips on one or both sides of the door. Another solution is to install offset hinges[6] that allow the door to swing out and away from the doorway, increasing the opening by two to three inches. If you cannot find offset hinges at your local home improvement store, contact your clinic or hospital occupational therapy (OT) or physical therapy (PT) department to find where you might purchase these and other helpful household adaptations.

129. **Keep doors swinging freely.** Keep hinges well oiled. If a door scrapes on the jamb or drags across a rug, plane the bottom to make it open and close more easily. To plane the bottom of a door without removing it, put a large piece of sandpaper on the floor under the door (padding it with newspaper if necessary to create a good contact surface) and then move the door back and forth a few times until it swings easily.

130. **Wind a few rubber bands around the largest part of the knob,** when turning a doorknob is difficult. The

rubber bands increase the diameter of the knob and make it easier to grasp. To increase the diameter even more, cover knobs with large or padded doorknob covers that are available at most hardware stores.

Under Lock and Key

131. **Adaptive key devices give better leverage.** Make turning keys easier with any number of adaptive devices that fit on your regular key. Hardware stores and home healthcare stores have different styles from which to choose. The EZ Key[7] can hold up to four keys. Be sure to try these devices first to see which works best for you.

132. **Mark important keys for easy identification.** Stop fumbling with keys. Put a piece of masking tape on your house or apartment key, or purchase rubber key covers, in different colors, shapes, and textures, so it's easy to identify the right key, even in the dark. Make it easier to locate the door lock at night by affixing reflective tape just above the key hole. Key covers and reflective tape are available at most hardware stores.

133. **Use fingerprint keypad locks to provide keyless access.** If you have difficulty managing keys, a fingerprint-activated door lock[8] might offer a solution. Program the lock to your fingerprint, and just a touch will unlock your door. The fingerprint door lock provides all the security of a conventional lockset, with the convenience of three different means of entry: conventional key, fingerprint, and PIN code. Keyless entries are available through a locksmith or home improvement store.

134. **Admit visitors with your garage door opener.** Stay safe behind locked doors yet avoid the effort of getting up and to the door when someone comes by keeping an extra garage door opener with you in the house. When

you want to let someone in, press the garage door opener from inside the house and let your guest in through the garage entrance.

135. Use a doorbell intercom. If you have trouble getting up and to the door in time to greet your visitor, have a qualified electrician install a doorbell-intercom system.[9] The system works like this: When a visitor rings the doorbell, every telephone in the house starts to ring (including cordless phones but not cell phones). When you answer the telephone, it works like an intercom, so that you can communicate with the person waiting outside. If you are on the phone when a visitor arrives, a call-waiting tone will sound to alert you. If you have a second doorbell at a side or back entrance to your house, the system can be wired with a distinct telephone ring for each doorbell. Some advanced systems even allow you to unlock the door from your telephone.

136. Use a wireless, remote door entry system to access your home without traditional keys. Press the battery-powered key fob, like those used in newer cars and trucks, and remotely activate your door lock from inside or outside the house (up to 164 feet away).[10] The locking mechanism may be mounted to any wooden door, operates cylinder and night-latch locks, and can be used in conjunction with traditional key locks for added security. For maximum security, the easy-to-program and reprogram fobs use a "rolling code" that changes each time the door is released. Comes with two key fobs, but up to ten may be added.

Railings, Stairs, and Grab Bars

137. Lead with your strong leg going up stairs, and with your weak leg going down. Remember, "Good leg to heaven, bad leg to hell."

138. **Signal others with flashing lights.** Save steps and attract the attention of someone who is in the basement by turning the light switch at the top of the stairs on and off a few times. The flashing lights will get the person's attention even if she has noisy equipment running or the volume on the TV cranked up.

139. **Install hand railings on both sides of a stairway,** so that you have support going up and down stairs. Basement stairs will be safer if you add abrasive rubber treads to each step. For added safety, paint the edge of the steps with luminous paint to make them more visible; alternate colors to avoid the chance of missing a step. To improve the lighting in the stairwell, use at least a 100-watt bulb.

140. **Use a portable tub suction bar as a helping hand.** If you need a little extra help getting up and down, a tub suction bar[11] may be just the thing. This portable handle has suction cups on each end activated by an easy-to-press lever. Simply place the suction cups on a smooth, dry surface, press the levers, and you instantly have a handle to lend you extra support. Use it at home where you need a helping hand, or carry it with you when you travel.

141. **Grab bars make getting up, down, and around easier** by allowing you to using leverage and larger muscle groups to assist you. Before installing grab bars, determine where they would provide the most help. A space the width of a clenched fist (about one and a half inches) should exist between the grab bar and the wall. Be sure to anchor the grab bars to the studs in the wall, so that they can withstand the pressure and weight of being used. Vinyl-covered hand grab rails are easier to grip and absorb less heat than metal; they are particularly useful in the bathroom and in outdoor areas. Grab bars are available at building supply and home health stores.

142. **Use a rail to help you get in and out of bed**, or up and down from chairs. The Smart-Rail™[12] is an innovative bed-assist rail designed for those requiring a little help for moving, standing, and/or transferring in and out of bed. Unlike fixed-style bed rails, Smart-Rail™ can unlock and pivot outward to provide better standing support with less reaching and twisting. More information is provided in the Resources section at the end of the chapter.

143. **Use a Super Pole System™[13] modular support to provide assistance with standing, transferring, or moving in bed.** The floor-to-ceiling pole is installed by simple jackscrew expansion. Available in a portable model, you can move the rail from place to place within your home, take it with you when you travel to visit the grandkids, or simply move it out of the way when it is not needed. Each portable model quickly secures and releases from a low-profile floor-mounted plate. Additional floor plates can be purchased to use.

Faucets and Sinks

144. **Install wrist blades on water faucets.** If you have separate controls for hot and cold water, consider installing wrist blades. Wrist blades are wide, wing-type handles that are operated by pushing with the forearm, wrist, or heel of the hand. They are available at most plumbing supply stores and hardware stores.

145. **Consider replacing bathroom faucets with kitchen faucets.** Turning water on and off is easier if you have a single lever arm to control the temperature and water pressure. Kitchen models generally have longer levers than bathroom models and are easier to use.

146. **Install a touchless faucet.** This is a wonderful aid for someone who finds it difficult to grasp or turn knobs, or

who perhaps forgets to turn off the water. A touchless faucet has an electric eye that senses the person's hands in front of it and turns the water on and off automatically. The faucet can be preset to a specific temperature to avoid scalding. Touchless faucets are available from plumbing contractors or home supply stores and may require professional installation.

147. Install a water wand if you have trouble with knobs. The EzFlo® water wand[14] is an inexpensive device designed for people who have trouble turning knobs on household sinks. A stick-like attachment hooks on your sink's faucet and is activated by a slight push. When you take your hand away, the water turns off.

148. Use a washcloth to help turn faucets on and off. If your hands are weak and you have trouble turning water faucets on and off, try using a washcloth to turn the knobs. You'd be amazed at how much easier the faucets are to operate.

The Bathroom

149. Try these adaptations for safer, easier use of your shower and bathtub:
- *Use a shower caddy*, a hanging basket that hooks over the shower head to keep soap and shampoo off the floor.
- *Use decorative non-slip tape or decals* in the tub or shower for improved traction.
- *Remove that slippery soap-film buildup* from rubber bath mats by periodically tossing them into a washing machine with soap and a little bleach or tea-tree oil (a greener alternative available in health food stores).
- *Have a seat while you bathe*; purchase one of the many inexpensive shower chairs available, or place a resin or webbed outdoor chair in the tub or shower.

- *Install grab bars in the shower and bathtub.* Never grasp towel racks or soap dish holders for support. Remember, grab bars must be securely anchored to wall studs.
- *Wrap rubber bands around the handle* of a hand-held shower nozzle to make it easier to hold and manage when your hands are soapy.
- *Keep your shower curtain sliding easily* by applying a light coat of petroleum jelly to the rod; rub off any excess with a paper towel.

150. **Improve your medicine chest and bathroom organization by doing any of the following:**
   - *Glue small magnets inside the medicine cabinet door* to hold nail files, cuticle scissors, and other metal objects.
   - *Use a spice rack placed at eye level to hold medications* or small articles that might easily be lost in a closet. They will be easier to spot, and you won't have to reach so far into the closet. (Check the clearance between the door and cabinet shelves before installing.)
   - *Put turntables on the bathroom counter,* in cabinets, or on closet shelves to make items easier to retrieve. You might also install pull-out shelves in lower cabinets.
   - *Reserve a drawer in the bathroom for clean undergarments.* That way, when you have finished showering, you have everything you need to start getting dressed.

151. **Raise your toilet seat.** If you find the height of standard toilet seats to be too low, purchase an adjustable portable toilet seat to increase the height by four to seven inches and make it easier to get on and off. Adjustable toilet seats are easy to attach to any toilet. Some portable seats provide armrests for added

support. Carry a tote bag and you can take the seat with you to safely use bathrooms away from home.

152. **Install a wall-mounted toilet**, at a level that is convenient for you. It leaves the floor space beneath free and easy to clean. Check with your local plumbing supply contractor for more information.

153. **Heat towels for instant warmth after bathing.** If you are affected by cold or damp, consider heating your towels. Microwave your bath towel and keep it warm in an insulated cooler while you bathe, or consider installing heated towel drawers—towels and blankets stored inside can instantly provide soothing warmth to sore joints and aching muscles. Look for towel warmers[15] at home improvement stores.

The Bedroom

154. **Keep a flashlight by the entrance to your bedroom.** Use it at night when you have turned off the light and need to illuminate the path to your bed. Then keep the flashlight on your nightstand so it will be handy if you need to get out of bed in the middle of the night.

155. **Choose the right bedding.** You will be more comfortable in bed if you choose the right bedding for your needs.
    - *Look for bed covers that provide warmth without weight*.
    - *Knitted sheets* are easier to put on the mattress because the corners stretch more easily than woven sheets.
    - *Satin sheets* or nylon or silk pajamas help you slide and turn over more easily. Do *not* wear slippery pajamas on slippery sheets however, or you may be so slippery that you fall out of bed.

156. Avoid undue weight or pressure on your feet and toes. If the bedding pressing on your feet and toes is painful or uncomfortable, try making a simple footboard from a piece of wood, or use a cardboard box. Place the wooden board or box at the end of the bed and drape the covers over it. The covers will lie across the footboard without touching your feet and toes. You can also purchase aluminum rails that will keep the covers off your feet. Ask about these at home health or bedding stores.

157. Consider repositioning your bed against a wall. If turning over or changing sleeping positions in bed is difficult, push the side of the bed up against the bedroom wall, and install a railing or grab bars at a height that makes turning easier. (Be sure to anchor the railing to a stud.)

158. Add bedrails to make getting in and out of bed easier. If moving in the early morning is hard, add bedrails made for young children (available in bedding or baby/toddler stores) to the side of the bed. The rail may give you better leverage and support when you try to stand up. Or, add Bed Handles,[16] a split rail that reduces twisting by giving you both right- and left-hand support handles.

159. An electric bed will give you a lift. If getting up and down is difficult, consider an electric bed that will help you rise and recline. Separate head and foot controls allow you to find the best and most comfortable position for you.

160. Organize bedroom closets for easy access.
- *Make top shelves and clothing rods the appropriate height* to reach without straining.
- *Keep items you wear and use often in the most easily accessible locations.*

- *Store items on shelves in transparent plastic containers* to make them easier to find and retrieve.
- *Label shoe boxes* with a brief description of the contents (e.g., "brown flats"). Use large letters on the edge of the cover to make locating shoes easier. Or, cut the end out of the box, keeping the cover intact, to easily see and retrieve shoes you want.

Furniture and Floor Coverings

161. Place chairs and couches approximately 17 inches off the ground so they're easier to get in and out of. Adjust the height of your furniture by adding or removing casters, or by placing measured blocks of wood under each leg until the desired height is achieved. Rubber height adjusters, made specifically for this purpose, may be purchased at furniture, bedding, or hardware stores.

162. Remove throw rugs to help prevent trips and falls. This will make navigating easier for those with trouble walking, or for those who use walkers, canes, and wheelchairs. If you must use a throw rug, purchase thin, rubber-backed entry door carpets or keep the rug from lifting or moving on the floor with a rubber mat (sold in carpet stores) or double-faced tape.

163. Apply felt pads to chair legs for ease of movement. When moving chairs becomes a burden, use felt pads on chair legs; they make sliding a chair on a wood or tile floor easier. These inexpensive pads are available at hardware stores or online.

Closets, Drawers, and Storage

164. Organize your closet floor using boxes with dividers. Plastic organizers from a discount store or cardboard boxes like those that hold liquor bottles will provide easily accessible storage for smaller items such as shoes. Cover the box with self-adhesive paper for a more finished look.

165. **Keep a laundry basket in every bedroom closet.** Laundry baskets are handy for holding and transporting laundry to the laundry room. Use light- and dark-colored baskets in each room to encourage everyone to sort their dirty clothes as they take them off. If lifting is difficult, purchase baskets with wheels that you pull behind you.

166. **Install a closet light.** Battery-powered lights which require no wiring are available at discount stores and mail-order companies. A little light makes it much easier to find things.

167. **Create a lower bar in a closet.** Purchase a closet organizer system or "do it yourself" by suspending a second closet rod from two equal lengths of rope hung from both ends of the existing closet bar. (The length of ropes will depend on how low you want the new rod to hang.) You'll double the hanging space for shorter items like blouses, shirts, and skirts.

168. **Lubricate drawer runs so they open easier.** Spray the runners with a dry silicone spray, available at hardware or building supply stores, or do what your grandmother used to do and rub a little candle wax or soap on the runners. Be sure to add drawer stops to prevent your easy-sliding drawers from pulling out and falling to the floor.

169. **Organize household items by storing like things together** and keeping them near the place in which they will be used. For example, sports equipment might be stored in the garage, sewing supplies and notions in the sewing-room closet, herbs and spices in the cupboard nearest the stove, and mittens and hats in a hanging shoe bag inside the coat closet. Keep family memorabilia

organized in individual cardboard boxes, labeling the boxes with the family member's name and the year. When the boxes are filled, they can be stored in the basement or attic.

170. **Shoe boxes are great for storing things** like cookie cutters, craft supplies, appliance cords, hair ribbons, and barrettes. Often shoe stores have empty boxes they're willing to give you. You can paint the box or cover it with an adhesive-backed paper so it's more attractive, then leave it out on a shelf or a countertop. If you store the boxes on a closet shelf, label the outside for easy retrieval.

171. **Store extra extension or appliance cords in empty toilet tissue and paper towel tubes.** The tubes are easy to grasp, and the cords stay neat and untangled. For easy identification, be sure to write the name of the appliance on the cord's tube.

172. **Store out-of-season items, like clothing and holiday decorations, in boxes that fit under the bed.** You can find plastic or cardboard boxes at discount department stores or wherever clothing organizers are found. Another solution is to use decorative storage cubes as tables, lamp or plant stands, and the like. Whatever you choose will save trips to the basement or attic storage areas.

Laundry

173. **Make your washer and dryer easier to use.** If you have trouble bending to get clothes in and out of the dryer, have the dryer raised to a comfortable height (perhaps six to eight inches higher) by setting it on top of wooden blocks or special risers available at hardware stores. Keep a reacher nearby for moving clothes from the washer to the dryer or from the dryer to the laundry basket; it will also come in handy if any clothes fall to the floor. Also, use a wheeled laundry cart instead of carrying regular laundry baskets.

174. Use a sheet of fabric softener to clean the lint trap in your washer or dryer. The treated sheets attract the lint, making it easier to remove; use the old sheet from the previous load.

175. Machine-wash small or delicate items in a pillowcase that you close with a rubber band. The clothes won't get snagged, and you won't have to reach deep inside the washing machine to find individual garments.

176. Reduce sorting and folding.
- *Purchase inexpensive sock sorters* (little colored rings you push the end of the sock through) and have your family use them before putting socks in the laundry basket; when socks are washed and dried, they will already be sorted and ready for the sock drawer. If you prefer, you can pin the socks together.
- *Maintain separate hampers for dark and light clothes.* Encourage family members to pre-sort their laundry by providing separate baskets or hampers for light and dark clothes.
- *Give yourself permission to NOT fold underwear.* Underwear is not seen, nor does it wrinkle in a way that prevents wearing; save energy and just toss them into the drawer unfolded.
- *Keep laundered bedding together* by first folding the pillow cases and bottom sheet and putting them aside. Then fold the top sheet length-wise and, when you're almost finished, put the pillow cases and bottom sheet inside, enveloping them in the top sheet. When you're ready to change the bed, all the sheets are in one compact package.

177. Avoid setting up a full-size ironing board for small jobs. Purchase a mini ironing board that you can set on a table or other surface set at the right height for you. Or, make one out of a piece of plywood—approximately 12 by 24 inches in size. Lay a towel over the board, cover with a pillow case, and you are ready to iron collars, shirt fronts, and other small jobs. Keep your mini board in a convenient place in the laundry room for quick access and no clean up.

178. **Stop lifting a heavy iron.** Purchase clothing that is either wrinkle-resistant or looks good wrinkled, and you will save hours of tedious labor. If you have shirts or clothing that really must be pressed, take them to your local laundry. They will do the heavy work for you at a nominal fee.

Housecleaning Details

179. **Wear rubber gloves to make it easier for weak hands to grasp objects.** They also help protect your hands from chemicals when cleaning and from the cold when handling frozen or refrigerated foods. To make the gloves easier to put on and take off, sprinkle a little cornstarch inside each one. If they're still difficult to remove, try holding your hands under cold water and then pulling them off. If one of the gloves gets a hole in it (usually the one for your dominant hand), keep the mate. The next time another dominant-hand glove wears out, turn the mate you saved inside out and you'll have a "new" pair of gloves. If gloves are too difficult to use, try slipping your hands into plastic bags; if necessary, secure around your wrist with a large rubber band.

180. **Vacuum instead of dust.** Get a lightweight canister vacuum, or an upright with an optional hand-held hose, turn the power to low, and vacuum instead of dusting. You will be amazed at how much time and effort this can save.

181. **Use a microfiber cloth to make cleaning easy.** Microfiber has a slightly tacky surface that attracts dirt and dust like a magnet. Use for dusting, for soaking

up spills, and polishing. Slip on a pair of microfiber gloves and run your hands over your blinds, furniture, bookshelves, chair rails, and carvings and just watch the dust disappear. For tougher cleaning jobs, moisten with water to improve the cloth's cleaning power. Microfiber cloths are available in the cleaning products section of your favorite department store.

182. Use an old sock as a dust cloth. Simply dampen the sock with dusting spray or furniture polish and slip it over your hand. This way your arms and shoulders do most of the work.

183. Use a lint roller. If, due to coordination or strength issues, it is difficult for you to clean, try using a lint roller to:
- *Clean lampshades* too delicate to vacuum.
- *Pick up pet hair* from furniture or floors.

A lint roller is easy to use, and the sticky surface picks up dust and dirt anywhere you can roll it.

184. Keep items from slipping with Dycem™. Cut a strip of this thin vinyl-like material (with a tacky, rubbery feel to it) and secure it around a pen, drinking glass, shaver, TV remote control, or other item, and the object will not slip out of your hands. Place Dycem under plates, bowls, and glasses to keep them from slipping away from you. Use one or two strips to help you open jars and cans, or use it to keep items from slipping away from you in the bathroom or on your nightstand.

Home health stores or hospital rehabilitation centers will help you locate this product. As an alternative, you might try using strips of waffle-style place mats or shelf liners readily available in kitchen departments.

185. Experiment with ways to carry items with you and keep your hands free. If gripping and holding items as you move them from place to place is painful, try:

- *Wearing an apron with pockets*; fill them with canned goods, cooking utensils, scissors, nails and a hammer, masking tape, and many other items.
- *A fishing or photographer's vest* is great for holding many small items.
- *Try using a drill holster* to hold a cordless phone or TV remote control.

You'll find these items at hardware, sport goods, or photographic stores.

186. **Use a wheeled cart.** Tea and utility carts, collapsible luggage carriers, and wheeled laundry carts all allow you to move heavy loads without carrying them. If you load a tea or utility cart with dishes, glasses, and silverware, you can set or clear the table in just one trip. Consider using a cart to move cleaning supplies or heavy items from room to room, or to move groceries from the car to the house.

    Collapsible box style carts may be stored in the trunk of your car for use whenever you need a little extra help carrying things—at the grocery store, mall, or other locations.

187. **Keep a small basket near the stairs** to hold items that need to be taken to rooms on a different floor of a multi-level house. You can collect the items throughout the day and easily carry them all at once. Specialty catalogs offer special baskets designed just for stairs.

188. **Keep items you use regularly in easy-to-reach locations.** If opening and closing drawers is difficult, bring your silverware and cooking utensils out of the dark. Try storing them in pretty containers on the countertop.

189. **Utilize easy-to-use containers.**
    - *Put detergent into a small, plastic pitcher* that is easier for you to pick up and pour than a heavy box of laundry or dishwasher detergent.

- *Pump bottles make dispensing easier*—everything from moisturizing lotion and liquid soap, to ketchup and salad dressing will dispense more easily in a pump bottle—no tops to unscrew or heavy bottles to lift.
- *Reuse empty liquid soap or lotion bottles,* or buy empty bottles at discount or bathroom supply stores.

190. **Use a child's play broom so you can sit to sweep the floor**; the broom is lightweight and easy to control. To avoid bending, use a broom-type sweeper. Try using a long-handled broom to sweep cobwebs off the ceiling.

191. **Polish chrome fixtures with rubbing alcohol.** It's quick, easy, and dries spot free.

192. **Make a washcloth "bracelet."** If you do not have a pair of rubber gloves when washing walls or windows, keep water from running down your arm by wrapping a washcloth around your arm, between wrist and elbow, and keep it in place with a thick rubber band.

Home Maintenance and Outdoor Chores

Outdoor Lighting

193. **Use a lemon on a string.** If you have a light bulb that turns on and off when you pull a string, make it easier to find and grasp the string by attaching an empty plastic lemon juice container (the kind that looks like a lemon) to the end. Or, use an old tennis ball; just punch two holes in the ball, run the string through, and tie tight.

194. **Wind holiday lights around an empty gift-wrap tube**, to prevent them from getting tangled. Insert the plug inside the tube and then wrap the lights around the outside. Secure the end of the light with a rubber band. You can wind several strings of lights around the same tube.

195. Lubricate the light bulb base before screwing into a socket. Put a dab of petroleum jelly or a spritz of a silicon-based lubricant, like WD-40, on the base of a light bulb and it will be easier to screw in and unscrew when it burns out.

196. Change outdoor lights all at the same time. Rather than getting out that heavy ladder and changing outdoor light bulbs when they burn out (usually at the most inopportune time or during inclement weather) change all your outdoor lights at one time and then annually thereafter. A good way to remember when to change the bulbs is to associate it with an annual date, like your birthday, anniversary, a holiday, or when you change the clocks ahead in the fall.

Tools

197. Store tools on a pegboard and use a marking pen to outline the space for each tool. Tools are at eye level, easy to reach, and you can tell at a glance if a tool is missing.

198. Purchase a foam kneeling pad (check the garden section) to cushion your knees, or use a partially filled hot water bottle to kneel on when washing floors or working in the garden.

199. Create a soft-grip on tool handles by wrapping with foam pipe insulation. Foam tubing is available in a variety of diameters. It's slit on one side so it's easy to install on the handles of household and outdoor tools like brooms, shovels, rakes, and mops. For indoor tools, keep the tubing in place with rubber bands or duct tape. For outdoor tools, wrap the handles with brightly colored electrical tape, so the tools are easier to find in the grass. You can find foam tubing at most hardware stores.

200. Add ergonomic handles to long-handled home and garden tools. Make it easier to grip and use brooms, shovels, rakes, and other tools without pain by adding ergonomic D- and T-grips mid-way up long handles.[17] Ask about them at hardware, garden, or home improvement stores. The Resources section at the end of the chapter lists more handy items.

201. **Keep nails handy when you're doing odd jobs around the house.** Wind a rubber band around the handle of your hammer close to the head and slip a few nails under the band, where they will be within easy reach when you need them.

202. **Mark the wall with moisture, to hang a picture and get in the right spot the first time.** Mark the spot on the wall with a moistened finger or sponge. Then, quickly hammer the nail in place before the area dries.

203. **Use a magnetic screwdriver to help you hold screws in place.** Touch the screw to the tool, and the magnetic field will hold it in place as you work—much easier than gripping a tiny screw and controlling the screwdriver at the same time. Be sure to keep magnetic tools away from your home computer and electronic media or your data may be scrambled.

204. **Use forearms for lifting heavy items.** If you must lift and move large, unwieldy, or heavy items, lifting straps[18] will help you to lift and carry with less stress on your body. Available at hardware or moving stores.

Yard Work

205. **Clip lawn or leaf bags to a fence with clothespins to make them easier to fill.** If the bags must stand alone, brace the bag upright and open by first filling a paper grocery bag with some of the lawn clippings; insert the partially filled grocery bag into the larger bag, and the lawn bag will be propped open. You might also stretch the leaf bag over a trash can to keep it open and

accessible; use one with wheels and it will be easier to move to your compost pile or yard waste collection site.

206. Use an old bracelet to remind you to turn off the water. If you have trouble remembering to turn off the sprinkler, try putting an old bracelet around your wrist to remind you that the water is on. When you turn the water off, leave the bracelet on the faucet, so it's ready to use the next time. The bracelet can save you steps and energy by eliminating extra trips to and from the faucet.

Gardening

207. Try alternate ways to garden. If you love the idea of home-grown vegetables but your body just won't allow you to get down and dirty anymore, try these alternatives:

- *Garden in raised beds.* If getting up and down is a challenge, try cultivating a raised garden bed. Build the flower bed out of lumber so that it is raised to about 34 inches or another comfortable height, fill with dirt, and plant. The raised bed wall makes a great place to sit while you tend your plantings, too. Be sure not to make the bed too wide to reach across.

- *Plant a trellis or container garden.* Exercise your green thumb by planting a few of your favorite things in a trellis or container garden. Choose a location on a low window ledge, balcony, walkway, or patio that is easy to reach and near a water supply. Plant in appropriate containers—clay pots are porous and allow excess water and salt to escape, yet you can place them inside more decorative pots, such as barrels, bushel baskets, window boxes, or hanging pots. Put the containers where you want them before you fill them with dirt; after filling, they will be too heavy to move. Most container-grown plants need to be watered more often than plants grown in the ground, so you might want to use self-watering pots or add moisture-absorbing pellets to reduce the need for watering. Check with your local green house, nursery, or garden center for more tips.

- *Garden indoors.* A sunny, south-facing window (or a shady spot supplemented with grow lights) can easily yield fresh healthy ingredients even in the dead of winter. Herbs in colorful containers can decorate a windowsill. An aquarium can act as a mini greenhouse, enveloping your plants in humidity and keeping watering chores to a minimum. You may be amazed at the multitude of edible plants, even citrus fruit, that can be grown indoors. Check with your local greenhouse or grower for the best varieties for indoor cultivation.

- *Plant preseeded "flower carpets."* If you want the beauty of flowers in your yard without a lot of work, try planting a "flower carpet." The seeds are embedded into a nutrient rich "carpet" that you just roll out onto soil loosened to a depth of three to four inches and raked smooth. Cover with an eighth-inch of soil to guard against strong winds, soak with a fine mist until saturated, and water daily until plants are three to four inches tall. (Seedlings appear in about one to two weeks, flowers in six to eight weeks.) For best results, purchase these preseeded carpets at nurseries, greenhouses, and garden mail-order companies.

208. Consult your local nursery or library about hardy plants and companion planting. Some flowers and vegetables, when grown together, help prevent damage from pesky insects and weeds. To make exercising your green thumb easier, ask a horticulturist to point out especially hardy plants and those that require less care.

209. Hang planters from a pulley rather than a hook. For easy watering of hanging planters, attach a rope to the hanger on the plant, thread the rope through the pulley, and pull the plant up. Tie the rope "figure-eight" style on two nails on the wall near the plant.

210. Protect your hands while gardening by purchasing gardening gloves that are one or two sizes too large. Then stuff foam or sponge-type padding in and around your fingers. When handling thorny plants, you might try using a quilted oven mitt.

211. Plant seeds without bending. One way to avoid bending while planting is to use a PVC pipe to guide seeds into the soil. Start with a three-and-a-half-foot section of one- or two-inch diameter pipe. Cut one end on the diagonal. Keeping the diagonally cut end of the pipe touching the ground, drop seeds down the pipe where you want the plants to grow. Cover the seeds using the end of the pipe or by dropping soil down the pipe. Another option is to fill a salt shaker or spice bottle that has a shaker top with seeds. After preparing the soil, simply shake the bottle over the areas you want to plant.

212. Sit on a stool or chair to work in the garden or flower bed and use well-made child-size rakes or shovels to work the soil. Some stools have wheels and storage compartments.

213. Mark your trowel for easy planting. When planting bulbs or other plants that need to be planted at a specific depth, purchase a trowel with pre-marked measurements or mark inches on your own tool with red nail polish. The markings will make it easier to dig to the proper depth.

214. Pull weeds when the ground is moist. Do your work after a rain, in the morning when the ground is still wet with dew, or after lightly moistening the ground with a garden hose. If you need a little extra help dislodging the roots, try an apple corer. Or, you might consider purchasing a long-handled weeding tool from a nursery or garden shop, so that you can weed without bending.

Garbage, and Trash Collection

215. **Recycle plastic store bags as wastebasket liners.** Put several empty grocery and discount store bags into the bottom of your wastebaskets, using one bag as the liner. When the liner bag is full, discard it and pull up another bag from the bottom of the wastebasket to use as the new liner. You'll save steps and recycle at the same time.

216. **Use smaller trash cans.** Many cities now provide large, wheeled trash cans designed for automated pick-up. If the large can that was delivered is too hard for you to handle, call your municipality to see if there is a smaller option. Of course, the smaller cans may mean more trips to the curb; you will have to balance this against the weight of the larger can.

217. **Use one wastebasket for recyclables and one for trash.** Help family members remember which is which by keeping recyclables on the right—it's "right" to recycle.

Winter Chores

218. **Use a plastic sled to slide trash cans to the curb.** When snow and ice impede getting the trash out, try placing bags or cans on a plastic sled and pull that to the curb. The sled will slide easily on the snow cover.

219. **Spray snow shovels so snow won't stick.** To make snow shoveling easier, apply an aerosol vegetable spray or furniture polish to the shovel so that the snow will slide off more easily.

220. **Use an ergonomically designed shovel or snow scoop for less strain on hands or back.** These can be purchased at most hardware stores.

221. **YakTrax®[19] provide extra traction on snow and ice.** Slip a pair of these steel-coil-wrapped rubber grips on your shoes or boots, and you will instantly have better traction and be less likely to slip and fall on snow and ice. They come in two styles: The Walker for walking/commuting, and the Pro, with an extra stabilizing strap for more active uses such as light hiking and running. Sizes range from extra small that will fit young people to extra large—women's 15.5+ and men's 14+. Check outdoor retailers for these and other similar devices.

RESOURCES

Remote Controls

1. **Universal Home Remote Control**

2. **Electronic Driveway Sensor**
   Smarthome
   16542 Millikan Avenue
   Irvine, CA 92606
   800-242 7329
   www.Smarthome.com

Lighting

3. **Lamp Switch Enlarger**

4. **Touch-sensitive Lamp Converters**
   Products for Seniors
   850 S. Boulder Highway, Suite 171
   Henderson, NV 89015
   800-566-6561
   www.ProductsForSeniors.com

5. **Light on Call**™
   548 Sunrise Highway
   West Babylon, NY 11704
   631-587-7414
   www. LightOnCall.com

Doors

6. **Offset Hinges**
   Dynamic Living
   95 W Dudley Town Road
   Bloomfield, CT 06002
   888-940-0605
   www.Dynamic-Living.com

7. **EZ Key**
   Arthritically Correct! Products
   P.O. Box 4047
   Stateline, NV 89449
   408-445-2011
   www.ArthriticallyCorrect.com

8. **Keyless Lock**

9. **Telephone Intercom**

10. **Wireless Remote Door Opener**
    Smarthome
    16542 Millikan Avenue
    Irvine, CA 92606
    800-242-7329
    www.Smarthome.com

Bed and Bath

11. **Tub Suction Cup Handle**
    Solutions
    P.O. Box 6878
    Portland, OR 97228
    800-342-9988
    www.solutions.com

12. Smart Rail™

13. Super Pole System™
Health Craft Products, Inc.
2790 Fenton Road
Ottawa, ONT, Canada K1T 3T78
888-619-9992
www.HealthCraftProducts.com

14. EzFlo® Water Wand
International Environmental Solutions, Inc./MEDFLO
2830 Scherer Drive North, Suite 310
St. Petersburg, FL 33716
800-972-8348
www.InternationalEnvironmentalSolutions.com.

15. Heated Towel Drawer
Smarthome™
16542 Millikan Avenue
Irvine, CA 92606
800-242-7329
www.Smarthome.com

16. Bed Handles
Bed Handles, Inc.
2905 SW 19th Street
Blue Springs, MO 64015
800-725-6903
www.BedHandles.com

Outdoors

17. Ergonomic Hand Grips
MOTUS, Inc.
P.O. Box 872
Winnipeg, MAN, Canada R3P 2S1
204-489-8280
www.Motus.mb.ca

18. Lifting Straps
Active Forever
10799 North 90th Street
Scottsdale, AZ 85260
800-377-8033
www.ActiveForever.com
www.ForearmForklift.com

19. YakTrax®
Yaktrax, LLC
9221 Globe Center Drive
Morrisville, NC 27560
866-YAKTRAX (925-8729)
www.YakTrax.com

CHAPTER 5

Managing
Mealtime Madness

The kitchen is often the busiest room in the house. It becomes a hotbed of activity when you're preparing and eating meals. Organizing your kitchen is but one part of streamlining the everyday activities that take place in this room—and meal planning, meal preparation, serving and eating a healthy diet are vitally important to people living with arthritis.

222. **Begin by building more time into your schedule to prepare and eat meals.** Make the kitchen or dining room a calm, low-stress environment by playing soft, relaxing music while you cook and eat.

223. **Do as much planning and preparation as possible while seated** at the kitchen table or at a stool pulled up to a countertop. If your energy or medication's effectiveness waxes and wanes, prepare meals when your energy level is high, and reheat food and serve it after you've had a chance to rest. When eating, sit close to the table and place all food and utensils within easy reach.

224. **Expect and encourage other family members to be part of meal preparation.** It's not anyone's sole responsibility to make dinner; give others tasks to do and accept their participation, even if you could do it faster and better. As they get older, and with practice, children will

learn how to fill the dishwasher correctly, wipe off the counters better, and sweep the floor properly. Be patient with children and adults; they will improve.

In our home, we had this mealtime rule: Everyone helps prepare dinner, and no one leaves the kitchen until everyone leaves. Even when our children were in elementary school, they understood our family rule. With each passing year, their level of involvement grew, the quality of their help improved, and the faster we were all out of the kitchen. The payoff has been watching my adult children, married with children and homes of their own, following our family tradition of preparing and eating meals together.

These ideas will make your kitchen more accessible, better organized, and safer. You'll also learn tips, techniques, and timesavers to save even more time and energy.

Making Your Kitchen User Friendly

Safety in the Kitchen

225. **Good lighting reduces fatigue and the risk of accidents.** Install under-cabinet lights in your kitchen workspaces. The lights, available from hardware and lighting-supply stores, come in a variety of sizes and styles.

226. **Keep a small flashlight in the kitchen.** A flashlight is not only handy in case the power goes out, but it makes it easier to find items in the back of deep cupboards.

227. **Consider replacing heavy dishes and cookware.** Replace heavy pottery mugs with porcelain, china, or insulated drinking cups. Lightweight dinner dishes are easier to lift and carry. Use lightweight cookware, gadgets with big cushioned handles, sharp knives, and stainless steel bowls to help you conserve strength and energy in the kitchen.

228. Choose a stove with controls on the front. Reduce reaching and make cooking easier by using a stove with controls on the front rather than the back. (If you have small children, you might want to remove the knobs when the stove is not in use.)

229. Tie a loop of fabric or cord around the handle, if opening the refrigerator door is tough. Avoid putting unnecessary strain on your hands and joints by using your forearms in the loop to pull the door open. The door is also easier to open if you place one or two strips of electrical tape across the bottom gasket; the appliance may be less energy efficient, but you'll need less strength to open the door.

230. Use rubber waffle-type pads to keep jars from slipping when opening. With a waffle pad in one hand, hold the jar; place a second pad on top of the jar, grip, and twist. Use this soft, grippy material wherever you need a little extra cushion, grip, or non-slip control—under drinking glasses, as a mat in the bottom of the sink, to keep things from sliding on a slippery surface—you will find many uses. You can find waffle grippers and shelf liners in the kitchen section of grocery and discount stores.

231. Use a cardboard carton to transport bottles to and fro. Fill a cardboard carton—the kind used for a six-pack of bottled drinks—with ketchup, mustard, salad dressing, and other items (even flatware and napkins), and carry them to the table all at once. You can store refrigerated items, even baby bottles, right in the carton to keep the bottles from tipping when you reach into the refrigerator.

Organizing Your Kitchen

232. Store items near the places where they're used, to save time and energy in the kitchen. Keep one set of measuring cups and spoons with the silverware and another near the stove. Keep coffee mugs near the coffee pot. Keep a measuring cup inside your flour or sugar canisters. Store microwave supplies, including microwave-safe containers and dye-free paper towels, in a cupboard close by.

233. **Store spices alphabetically in a drawer or spice rack;** spices will be easier to find and use than in a high cupboard. To maintain freshness, keep them away from a heat source like the stove or refrigerator.

234. **Remove the magnetic door catches on difficult-to-open cabinet doors.** Install easy-to-grasp hardware, like U-shaped handles, on the outside of cabinets. If doors are too hard to use, remove them; if you do not want to see what is inside, hang fabric curtains over the opening. Check building supply stores for handles that work best for you.

235. **Add additional, easily accessible storage space.**
    - *Install hooks under kitchen cabinets.*
    - *Hang pots and pans* by installing a peg board or hanging pot rack on the wall or ceiling.
    - *Hang small gadgets and pot holders* on the side of the refrigerator using magnetic hooks.
    - *Store frequently used utensils in decorative jars* on the countertop.
    - *Store baking pans and trays in a cupboard equipped with vertical dividers*. Standing pans between dividers eliminates the need to lift several to get to the one you need—usually on the bottom. Check with a carpenter or kitchen cabinet supplier about installing the dividers.

236. **Store flour, sugar, and coffee in lightweight containers** with handles and easy-to-remove lids. Keep them on the counter to avoid having to reach for and lift heavy containers, and keep a measuring cup inside, where it is handy and easy to use.

237. **Store cheeses and lunch meats together**, so that all the fixings for a sandwich are in one container or bag. If you do not want the meat to touch the cheese, use a divided storage container or two individual plastic bags that you can put together in one.

238. **Roll bottles and jars on the countertop, instead of shaking them to mix ingredients.** It is easier on the hands.

239. **Freeze extra cookies.** Each time you bake cookies, freeze a few so you'll always have an assortment to serve whenever company arrives.

240. **Mix cookie dough with just one beater on your mixer;** doing so keeps the dough from climbing up the beaters. If traditional cookie cutters are hard to use, try using a metal, glass, or hard-plastic tumbler instead; dip the tumbler in flour before each use so the dough won't stick.

241. **Cover your hand with a clear plastic sandwich bag before you grease baking pans**, make meat loaf, or roll cookie dough. You might also use inexpensive, disposable gloves available at drug or hardware stores (be sure they are unpowdered), or use the empty butter wrapper to keep your hands from getting greasy while greasing the pan.

242. **Freeze leftovers as complete dinners.** Put serving-size portions of leftover food on a microwaveable plate and cover first with plastic wrap and then with aluminum foil and freeze. (The double wrap will help keep the food from becoming freezer burned.) When you're ready to eat, remove the wrappings, cover with another microwaveable plate, and reheat the meal in the microwave. If you don't have or prefer not to use a microwave, conserve energy and save on clean-up time by heating small amounts of leftovers, wrapped

in single-serving aluminum foil packages, side-by-side in a covered frying pan containing an inch of water. Only one pan to wash!

Tools, Small Appliances, and Equipment

Kitchen tools have come a long way in the last few years in becoming simpler, more specialized, and, most importantly for someone with arthritis, more ergonomically designed to work with your body and cause less pain. If the tools in your kitchen have been around awhile, consider some of the following; unless otherwise indicated, you will find these items in fine kitchen stores or in any well-stocked kitchen department.

243. **Use a slow cooker to prepare meals early in the day**, when your energy is usually at its best. Plus, there's no standing at the stove, hot pots to handle, or major clean-up to do at the end of the day.

244. **Turntables make a variety of items easier to reach.** Use one inside your refrigerator, and others in kitchen and bathroom cabinets to bring desired items within reach. Put one on the kitchen counter or in the middle of the dining room table to make it easier to reach napkins, condiments, and other items.

245. **Cook in an electric frying pan or wok**, so that you can sit at the kitchen table while you cook. Less clean up too.

246. **With PurrfectOpener™,[1] bottles, caps, and cans open easily.** If your hands aren't working like they used to, the multiple openings of the PurrfectOpener™ will fit over bottle and pill caps and give extra leverage for opening. It also has a handy tail for opening milk bottles, pop tops and pull tabs; ears to pierce safety seals; and even openings for splitting pills. Use the magnetic back to keep the opener affixed to your refrigerator or

stove and within easy reach. Find this or a similar product at drug stores or order online.

247. **Use a Universal Opener[2] to open packaging with ease.** If you have difficulty opening bags, boxes, cans, containers, and other packaged items, the Ableware® Open-It™ Universal Opener is a necessity for you. This multifunctional device features a protected blade for opening bags and boxes, a "poke" for opening container lids and making holes in drink boxes, and a "hook" for opening pull tabs on cans. It can also be used for peeling oranges and opening envelopes or vacuum-sealed packages.

248. **Replace hard to grip utensils with large, cushioned-handle versions.** To get an easier grip on cooking, replace old potato peelers, spatulas, whisks, and others with modern gadgets that have large, cushioned handle grips. OXO International[3] kitchen products, sold in the kitchen, garden, and housewares sections of department and grocery stores, include a number of specialty and hard-to-find cooking utensils (cookie scoop, spice grinders) and other easy-grip products and tools for home and garden.

249. **Use an automatic jar opener.** If you are always asking someone else for help in opening jars, an automatic jar opener will help you. The OXO Good Grips i-Series Jar Opener[4] is unique in that it uses the jar gripper in combination with an innovative base pad that holds the jar in place, improves leverage, and reduces the force necessary to open most jars—from small containers of condiments to large tubs of mayonnaise. To use, simply place the non-slip base pad under your jar to keep it secure on the countertop, slide the jar opener over the jar lid to engage the riveted stainless steel teeth, and twist counter-clockwise to loosen. The wide, contoured handle is non-slip to improve turning leverage. The

non-slip base pad attaches securely to the jar opener for storage. The jar opener is dishwasher safe; the pad may be hand washed if necessary. For more information on this and other OXO products, check the Resources section at the end of the chapter.

250. **Try angled measuring cups to make measuring easier.** Avoid having to lift a measuring cup to accurately gauge the contents by using angled measuring cups from OXO.[5] Available in four-cup, two-cup, one-cup, and a mini size that measures small amounts up to four tablespoons, all are marked so amounts can be accurately read while the cup sits on the counter.

251. **Use an automatic can opener.** Automatic can openers like the One Touch™ hand-held or the Black & Decker Spacemaker™[6] that mount under your cabinets, make opening cans much easier on stiff, sore hands. Visit your local kitchen or home store and ask to try a few to see which works best for you.

252. **Ergonomically designed knives lessen the strain on your hands** and that allow you to use your entire arm when cutting foods. Look for a knife with a large handle that allows you to "saw" back and forth when cutting.

253. **A rocker knife and cutting board chops and dices with ease.** If you find chopping and dicing to be a pain in the wrist, consider getting a rocker knife. Used by native Alaskans for centuries, the ULU rocker knife[7] has a large, easy-to-grip wooden handle that sits directly above the blade, so that the knife and hand become one, increasing dexterity and leverage, making fine cuts simple, and chopping easier. Use the knife alone, or make it even easier to cut and keep the items being chopped contained by pairing the knife with the walnut and birch cutting bowl, designed to fit the curved blade of the ULU knife. You can also turn

the cutting bowl over and use the back for a flat cutting surface.

254. **The Prep Taxi™[8] safely carries food from cutting board to pan or bowl.** The Prep Taxi™ is a unique scoop that allows you to slice, dice, and chop food in preparation for cooking and, with one easy motion, safely move what you have chopped to your cooking pan or bowl. Its six-inch wide, flat, stainless steel mouth holds up to three cups, and its one-inch high sides help prevent spills.

255. **Use a pastry blender to mix foods or stir and separate ground meat.** Its large, thick handle makes it easier to use than a fork or mixing spoon.

256. **Create a lower work surface** to use while seated by setting a cutting board or cookie sheet over an open drawer at the height that works for you.

257. **Make kitchen clean-up easier by soaking pans with a little baking soda in the water.** Let it sit a while, and the cooked-on food will easily wash away. If you need a little more oomph, try a Black and Decker Powered Kitchen Scrubber.[9] Battery-powered, weighing less than eight ounces and with an easy-to-hold angled grip, this fully submersible scrubber will power away stuck-on food. It comes with an assortment of attachments for light- to heavy-duty jobs; you might even want to buy an extra for the bathroom. Look for power hand scrubbers at hardware or home improvement stores.

Grocery Shopping

258. **Cut out coupons with ease, despite limited hand strength:**
    - *Try using a lightweight, rotary paper trimmer.* Great for cutting coupons, photos, scrapbook materials, even lightweight fabrics for quilts, the cutting edge is

mounted in the guide so you always get a nice straight edge. To use, simply lift the guide, slide your paper or craft materials underneath, close the guide, and move the sliding cutter across your materials; it cuts strips as little as three-quarters of an inch wide. Several sizes are available for home, office, or craft uses at fabric, craft, scrapbook, or office supply stores.

- *Make cutting easier with a self-opening loop scissors.*[10] A simple squeeze is all that is needed to cut through paper and lightweight plastic; release, and the scissors reopens on its own so you are always ready for the next cut. This scissors may be used with either the right or left hand.

- *Push-down scissors cut without gripping.* Just place this cutter[11] on the table, put what needs to be cut under the blade, push down with your hand, and paper or fabric is cut.

259. **Make a master grocery list.** Reduce the need to write a grocery list by creating a diagram of the store and listing the food categories for each aisle (some stores offer a preprinted map). Then, make a master grocery list (the computer is handy for this) of items you purchase regularly, in the order you find them in the store. Each week, hang a copy on the refrigerator and simply circle needed items; by the end of the week, the map becomes your shopping list. This system saves time and energy and is especially helpful if someone who is unfamiliar with the store has to shop for you.

260. **Prioritize your grocery list, marking the most important items.** If you run out of energy at the store, you'll be sure to get the items you most need. Recycle used envelopes as grocery lists and coupon carriers. Clip the envelope to the refrigerator, writing your list on the back and putting your coupons inside. Then, clip the envelope to the grocery cart to keep the coupons handy

and your hands free. If someone helps you shop for groceries, save box tops and labels of the packaged foods you need in the envelope; this will help them select the right product, brand, and size.

261. Shop when the store is least busy. Not only is it easier to shop when you do not have to cope with aisles full of shoppers, but often you can get special services not available during busier times of the day. For example, the person at the deli counter might dice your onions and place them in a plastic bag, or the cashier might break the seals of hard-to-open jars. According to a survey by a national grocery association, Tuesday is the least busy day of the week. However, call your favorite store to find out the days and times that are quietest.

262. Inquire about special services to make your life easier. Some grocery stores offer special services to help shoppers select and pick up the items they need. Smaller neighborhood stores may provide home delivery—simply call in your "order" and, for a fee, they will deliver groceries to your home. Larger chain stores may not deliver, but they sometimes maintain a list of companies that offer pick-up and delivery service from their store. If stores near you do not deliver, you may be able to call ahead and request that the store assemble a few items that you need and have them ready for you to pick up at a specified time. If you would like assistance in getting to and from your car, ask about having a store employee meet you at your car. Call stores in your area to ask about the services you would find most helpful, then patronize those that provide these services.

263. Consider grocery shopping online. Online grocers like NetGrocer.com and PeaPod.com offer delivery to your door of basics, organics, and hard-to-find items. For a more complete list of firms and services, search "online grocery" on the Internet.

264. Let children help you shop. Depending on their ages, enlist your children in finding and retrieving items from shelves. You might say, "Find the box with white flowers on it, the twelve-ounce bottle of salad dressing, and the spaghetti sauce with mushrooms and garlic." It takes more time, but it's a great learning experience for the kids, while it helps you save energy.

265. Use a scooter to conserve energy while shopping. Many stores offer motorized shopping scooters or wheelchairs as a convenience for their customers. Do not be embarrassed to use them if it makes your shopping trip easier. You can collect items in the basket that's attached to the front of the scooter.

266. Wear a glove with leather on the palm and fingers to help you grasp glass bottles and metal cans. The glove will also keep your hands warm while handling cold foods.

267. Purchase food that is already diced, sliced, cut, or shredded. Buy veggies already cut and peeled and ask to have large, heavy packages of meat, cheese, and the like divided into smaller, more manageable portions. On particularly difficult days, let the deli prepare dinner for you—buy barbecued chicken, a salad, and a vegetable, and you will have a healthy meal ready to eat when you arrive home.

268. Purchase nonperishable food items in advance. Shopping can leave you weary, so don't do it any more often than necessary. Stock up on nonperishable items; buy in bulk every month or two at direct warehouse stores like Sam's Club, Costco, and Wal-Mart. Even local grocery stores are an option; ask about the price of case lots of frequently used nonperishable items; doing so may save you considerable time, energy, and money.

269. Ask the bagger not to fill your bags too full. Spread out the items into more bags that will weigh less. Ask that all frozen or perishable foods be put into one bag; if you are sore and tired when you arrive home, you only need to empty one bag immediately—the others can wait.

270. Use rubber bag handles[12] to ease strain on hands. If you have trouble gripping or holding on to traditional bag handles or they simply hurt your hand, consider using a folded washcloth or rubber bag handle to cushion your grip. Small enough to stow in your purse or glove compartment, they are ready in an instant to wrap around and soften the grip of grocery bags, shopping bags, even paint cans. The cushioned rubber grip is soft and easy to hold. Check with your local discount or hardware store for availability.

Meal Planning and Preparation

271. Try planning meals one week at a time. Prepare your grocery list at the same time, and you'll eat better, save money, and make fewer trips to the grocery store for necessary ingredients. Once you have planned your meals, post the menu where everyone can see it; note recipe and cookbook pages on the list so that any family member can chip in and help when needed.

272. Prepare ahead and freeze meals when you can. You might prepare parts of meals in advance or make double recipes and freeze the leftovers for a day when you do not feel like cooking.

273. Get family members involved in meal planning. Allow each member, including children, to plan meals and make or dictate a list of the ingredients needed. At holiday time, try baking with friends in assembly-line fashion. Have everyone bring a favorite recipe and necessary ingredients.

274. Sit while preparing food. Rest and reduce undue stress on your joints by sitting on a tall stool while preparing meals. Some come with backs for added support, and wheels to allow you to roll easily from countertop to stove. A pneumatic "drafting" stool version will adjust to the proper height with just the touch of a lever. Inquire at your local office supply store.

275. Mount an adjustable mirror over the stove, to make it easier to cook while seated. Angle it so you can more easily see into pots and pans on the stove.

276. Keep a large bowl or small wastebasket on the counter during meal preparation. Avoid unnecessary bending by lining a large bowl or small wastebasket with a recycled plastic bag and toss in vegetable peels, empty packages, cans, and other waste as you work. When you're finished cooking, discard everything at once.

277. Keep recipe cards where you can see them by inserting them between the tines of a fork. Place the fork in a glass, and your recipe card will stay clean and easy to read.

278. Store plastic wrap in the freezer to make it easier to use. When it warms up it will regain its cling.

279. Peel and cut vegetables ahead of time. Keep carrots, celery, and other cut vegetables fresh and crisp by putting them in a container with an ice cube or two, and store in the refrigerator. Place in zipper-type bags, and a healthy snack is always ready to grab on the go.

280. Bake casseroles and pies on an aluminum-foil lined baking sheet, shallow roasting pan, or jelly roll pan. The dishes will be easier to lift, and the larger outer pans will catch any spill-over, eliminating oven cleaning.

281. Use a cool-to-the-touch, handled colander inside your cooking pan. Cook pasta or potatoes in the colander, and when done, simply lift it out, drain, and serve. You can use the same method to cook vegetables, or you might want to consider a steamer. Purchase a cool-handled colander or steamer wherever cookware is sold.

282. Make broiler pans easier to clean with a cup of water poured into the bottom portion of the pan before cooking. The water keeps drippings from being baked on and eliminates smoke during cooking. If food does stick to pots or pans, add baking soda and water while the pan is still warm, let cool, and clean up is easy.

283. Use frozen bread to make sandwiches. It's easier to spread peanut butter, jelly, margarine, and other spreads if the bread is frozen. Frozen bread doesn't tear, and it defrosts so quickly that by the time you finish the task and get to the table, the sandwich will be ready to eat. Whenever possible, select whipped butter and cream cheese; these products are much easier to spread than traditional varieties.

284. Moisten your fingers first when you pick up and hold eggs. Place eggs in an empty egg carton when carrying them from the refrigerator to a work area, or take the whole carton from the refrigerator to the counter while you work. Beating eggs is easier if you use a wire whisk or pastry blender, or, break the eggs into a jar, screw the lid on tightly, and shake.

285. Separate eggs with a small kitchen funnel placed over a measuring cup. Break the egg into the funnel; the white will slip neatly and easily into the measuring cup, while the yolk stays in the funnel. You can also purchase an egg separator, designed to fit over a standard measuring cup. If you do not have either:

- *Crack eggs on the rim of an empty bowl,* the thinner the rim the better. If pieces of the shell fall into the bowl, retrieve them by using a larger piece of the eggshell to scoop under the broken piece; the piece will be attracted to the shell and you can scoop it out easily.

- *Drop it!* For those with limited fine motor control, hold the egg about 10 or 12 inches above an empty bowl and drop it; the egg will break in two, making the shell easy to remove.

Serving Meals

Making or Using Simple Adaptive Devices at Mealtime

286. **Use a spoon as a knife.** If you have weakness in your hands, try using a spoon as a knife. The bowl of the spoon fits in the palm of your hand and the long smooth handle acts as your knife blade.

287. **Use a pour spout to make pouring oil easier.** Add a pour spout, like bartenders use, to oil bottles— no more caps to twist off and on—just lift and pour. The pour-spout is a standard bartender's tool that you will find at kitchen stores; some, like the OXO wine stopper/pourer, close to preserve freshness between pours.

288. **Run hot water over a plastic lid to make it more pliable** and easier to put on a container.

289. **Attach small casters or wheels to the underside of a cutting board.** Use the adapted cutting board as a trivet or to move heavy pots or dishes from one place to another. As an alternative, purchase a rolling plant-pot "trivet" at garden shops; these are used to move heavy planters, but will work with heavy bowls and pots too.

290. Reduce spills with a spill-proof travel mug.[13] Are you finding it hard to hold onto your coffee mug? If you're spilling more than you're drinking, a spill-proof travel mug might be the solution. OXO offers a vacuum-seal travel mug that won't leak, even upside down. It keeps your beverage hot or cold up to seven hours, at home or on the road. Available at kitchen and travel stores or contact OXO for a location near you.

RESOURCES

Openers

1. **PurrfectOpener**™
   B.A. Maze, Inc.
   c/o R. Mazur
   43311 Joy Road
   Canton, MI 48187
   800-708-6736
   www.PurrfectOpener.com

2. **Open-It**™ **Universal Opener**
   Maddak Inc.
   661 Route 23 South
   Wayne, NJ 07470
   973-628-7600
   www.Maddak.com

Kitchen Tools and Gadgets

3. **Ergonomic and Cushioned-handle Kitchen Tools**

4. **Automatic Jar Opener**

5. **Angled Measuring Cups**
   OXO International
   75 Ninth Avenue, 5th Floor
   New York, NY 10011
   800-545-4411
   www.oxo.com

6. **Home Appliances**
   Black & Decker
   101 Schilling Road
   Hunt Valley, MD 21031
   800-544-6986
   www.BlackandDecker.com

7. **ULU Knife and Cutting Board**
   Dynamic Living
   95 West Dudleytown Road
   Bloomfield, CT 06002
   888-940-0605
   www.Dynamic-Living.com.

8. **Prep Taxi**
   Chef's Planet®
   2120 E. Rose Garden, Suite E1
   Phoenix, AZ 85024
   602-906-3600
   www.ChefsPlanet.com

9. **Powered Kitchen Scrubber**
   Black & Decker
   101 Schilling Road
   Hunt Valley, MD 21031
   800-544-6986
   www.BlackandDecker.com

Cutting

10. **Loop Scissors**
    North Coast Medical, Inc.
    18305 Sutter Boulevard
    Morgan Hill, CA 95037-2845
    800-235-7054
    www.BeAbleToDo.com

11. Push-Down Scissors
Sammons Preston
P.O. Box 5071
Bolingbrook, IL 60440-5071
800-323-5547

12. Baggy Buddy
P.O. Box 4269
Ft. Lauderdale, FL 33338
www.BaggyBuddy.com

13. Travel Mug
OXO International
75 Ninth Avenue, 5th Floor
New York, NY 10011
800-545-4411
www.oxo.com

CHAPTER 6

Looking Good, Feeling Better

How you look has an impact on how you feel. Wearing comfortable and stylish clothing and being well groomed lifts the spirits in a way that a pair of old blue jeans and a faded, over-sized sweatshirt never could. In this chapter, you'll find ways to streamline grooming and dressing, so that you will have more time and energy to pursue other daily activities.

291. **Alter the order of your morning rituals.** Experiment and discover a sequence that works for you with regard to taking your medication, showering, grooming, eating, and dressing. Always give yourself more time to complete morning tasks. You may want to get up earlier than other family members, so that you don't feel rushed if you're trying to be ready at the same time as everyone else.

292. **Gather all your clothing items together before you start to dress** you'll save steps and time.

293. **Sit on the bed or in a sturdy chair with armrests when you dress.** If your balance is unsteady, you may also want to sit when you do your hair, shave, or apply makeup.

294. **Use a combination of store, catalog, Internet, and TV shopping** to find the stylish clothing and accessories you want.

Grooming

295. Brush teeth with an angled or long-handled tooth-brush. If brushing your teeth is difficult because you can't raise your hand or arm comfortably, purchase an angled toothbrush; lengthen the handle of your tooth-brush with a ruler, tongue depressor, or a long wooden spoon; or bend the handle of a pliable toothbrush your-self by running hot water over it for 60 seconds and gen-tly bending it to the desired angle. You might also find a battery-powered or sonic toothbrush easier to hold and use. There are many types to choose from; some have long, built-up handles for easier gripping, some are cord-less, and some have dual motion—up and down, and side to side. When purchasing a powered toothbrush, be sure to hold it in your hand, turn it on, and see how heavy and maneuverable it is before you buy.

296. Flosbrush® makes flossing easy. If it is hard for you to hold and maneuver regular floss, this handy flosser on a toothbrush-style handle, with an angled neck and compact head, will help you to floss even your back teeth with more control. The flosser comes in a variety of floss choices—premium, shred-resistant, mint waxed, and even a fruit-flavored version that will appeal to children. Ask about this product at a drug-store near you.

297. Use a hand-held or adjustable-height shower nozzle. If you need to shower sitting down, or if bending to bathe children or pets is difficult, consider attaching a hand-held or adjustable-height shower head to your shower. Hand-held nozzles come in a variety of styles that usually screw into the existing shower connection without any professional help. Adjustable-height shower heads which may require professional install-tion, have a bar that the shower head slides up and down on, so that you can adjust the head to the proper height of the user. You will find additional shower options at home improvement stores.

298. **Substitute a wash mitt or soft sponge for the usual washcloth.** Sponges are usually easier to use if your hands are weak.

299. **Telescoping mirrors let you sit down when grooming.** Telescoping mirrors clamp to the side or sit on top of your vanity; they feature adjustable, swivel-type necks that may easily be moved to various positions. Look for one with a double-sided mirror—one side is a regular mirror and the other side is magnified, making it perfect for makeup application or shaving. You might also consider installing mirrored tiles at various heights on the bathroom walls.

300. **Pop-up tissues are easier to grasp** than the kind that lie flat in the box.

301. **End shaving with electrolysis.** If you have heavy leg or underarm hair, and it is difficult for you to hold or maneuver a razor, consider investing in electrolysis. Once the hair is removed, you will have only smooth skin, no more shaving, and no more nicks, cuts, or razor rash.

302. **Trim your toenails with long-handled scissors.**[1] To give you better leverage and make cutting easier, look for scissors with serrated, stainless steel blades and long handles (8½ inches) that angle upward. Molded finger and thumb grips help hold the scissors securely in your hand. Look for these and other long-handled personal care products at drug or home health stores, or see the Resources section at the end of the chapter.

303. **Use a hands-free stand to aid styling your hair.** If you have difficulty blow-drying your own hair, you may like Active Forever's Pro-Styling Stand.[2] With a stable base and moveable neck, you can easily insert your

blow dryer handle into the cushioned holder at the top, adjust the bendable neck to fit your height, and style your hair by simply turning your head. The Pro-Styling Stand is perfect for people who have trouble holding a dryer or have limited arm strength. Some assembly is required. For more information, see the Resources section.

Dressing Tips and Aids

304. **Each night, select your clothing for the next day.** This will not only save time and energy in the morning, but if you need assistance with buttons or zippers, you will be able to enlist the aid of a family member before he leaves the house.

305. **Choose what you wear based on the day's activities.** If you plan on swimming, for example, choose an easy-on, easy-off outfit with few buttons, zippers, or ties. If you will be traveling, wear something that is a little looser, in a slippery fabric that makes it easier for you to change positions or get in and out of an uphol-stered seat.

306. **Dress in front of a mirror.** Seeing as you are doing can help uncooperative fingers do their work, and you are less likely to miss any buttons.

307. **Alleviate the discomfort of bra straps with silicone cushions.** If wearing a bra aggravates or causes pain in your neck, shoulders, or arms, silicone bra strap cush-ions[3] may help. The three-and-a-half-inch–long, hypoallergenic cushions slip nearly invisibly under straps, distributing weight more evenly while holding bra straps in place more securely. You may find these cushions helpful to redistribute the weight of your purse or keep shoulder straps from slipping off nylon outerwear.

308. Use a dressing stick. If you have pain in your shoulder, a dressing stick will extend your reach and may help you to pull on shirts and jackets without discomfort. Make your own using the hook end of a wire hanger or screw a small cup hook into the end of a dowel.

Shopping for Clothing

General Shopping Tips

309. Shop, don't drop. To make your next trip to the mall more manageable, keep these time- and energy-saving tips in mind:

- *Shop weekdays and early mornings.* Shop at less busy times, and you will avoid crowds and long lines.
- *Check out the floor plan and plot your course.* You can do this online or, if you don't have a computer, ask at the service desk for directions or a map of the store(s).
- *Call ahead.* If you know exactly what you want, call ahead and ask the store to have it ready for you when you arrive. Some stores will let you pay for items with a credit card over the phone, making it possible for someone else to pick up your purchases.
- *Find a fitting room with a chair.* This gives you an opportunity to rest a little. If no chair is available, ask a sales person to get one for you, or ask if you can take the clothes home "on approval" and try them on at your leisure. Another option is to shop with a friend who wears the same size as you do; have your friend try on the clothes you like and, if they fit your friend, you know they are likely to fit you. Just be aware however, that your coloring may be different from your friend's, and that will have an effect on how the clothes look on you.

- *Make purchases in less busy departments.* To conserve time and energy while shopping at a department store, pay for your purchases in a low-traffic area such as the men's or children's department; in drugstores, pay at the cosmetics or photo counter for faster service.
- *Don't carry a lot of bags.* Use a shopping cart or borrow or rent a baby stroller to wheel around with your purchases. Ask for assistance to get purchases to your car, or keep a folding cart in your trunk. If you do need to carry multiple or heavy bags any distance, keep a washcloth handy to wrap around the handles and cushion the strain on your hands.
- *Take breaks.* Stop for a drink in the food court or buy a magazine and sit down in a store or mall lounge to read a while. Resting from time to time will help you to shop longer.

Choosing the Right Clothing

310. **Look good without a lot of effort.** When choosing clothing, keep the following easy dressing tips in mind:
   - *Wear lightweight fabrics.* Garments made from heavyweight fabrics may actually tire you out just putting them on. Purchase lighter-weight clothing, and wear layers under a jacket or sweater for added warmth.
   - *Select wool garments lined with a satiny fabric* so they pull on and off easier. If you have unlined slacks, purchase lightweight silk or nylon pant liners to wear underneath.
   - *Nylon underwear makes pulling pants up and down easier* than wearing cotton underwear.
   - *Clothing that opens in the front is easier to put on and take off* than garments that open in the back. Partially button shirts, and then slip them over your head. If you struggle to get buttons through a buttonhole, make the buttonhole slightly larger by slip-

ping an emery board into the opening and sliding it back and forth the length of the buttonhole a few times. If you choose clothing that pulls over your head, make sure it has enough stretch to make it easy to get on and off.

- *Zippers are easier to use than buttons.* When fingers are stiff and uncooperative, however, it can be hard to grasp small zipper pulls. If you struggle with zipper pulls, attach a key ring, charm, or large cushioned zipper pull that you can grasp with your whole hand. You will find large zipper pulls in luggage departments; these are more appropriate for outdoor jackets, luggage, and purses however.
- *Wear clothing with elastic waistbands.* Avoid zippers and buttons altogether by wearing elastic-fit pants in stretchy fabrics that are easy to pull up and down.
- *Choose clothing one size larger.* Clothing that is too tight may actually make you feel tired. If you purchase garments one size larger than you normally wear, clothing will go on and off easier and be more comfortable to sit in. Queen-size pantyhose are easier to pull up and down than regular sizes.

311. **Buy more than one.** When you find a garment you like, in a style and size that fits, purchase several in various colors. This will save you time and energy in the long run.

312. **Look sharp with preknotted zipper ties.**[4] If you have difficulty tying a necktie, try adjustable, preknotted zipper ties (designed for adults). Zipper ties are worn by putting the loop over the head, under the shirt collar, and then pulling downward.

313. **Wear shawls instead of coats.** Unless the weather is terribly cold or inclement, consider wearing a shawl instead of a coat if the pain and stiffness in your hands and shoulders makes it difficult to button, zip, or put your arm in sleeves.

Hosiery and Footwear

314. Wear shoes with proper support. If you take care of your feet, your whole body will thank you for it. Footwear with proper support not only cushions every step, but it promotes proper posture and thus relieves pain. Companies such as Merrell, Keen, and Chaco[5] make shoes, even flip-flops, with durable, supportive foot beds that pamper your feet and stand the test of time. Visit a shoe store with expert fitters who will measure your feet and recommend the best choices for you. You may pay a little more, but it is worth it. For more information on special shoes, see the Resources section at the end of the chapter.

313. Buy shoes that are comfortable and fit properly:
- *Make sure there's a quarter to half-inch of space between the end of your longest toe and the end of the shoe.* To check, press with your thumb at the end of the shoe; you should not feel your toe under your thumb.
- *Make sure you can wiggle all of your toes* comfortably inside the shoe.
- *Feet swell during the day*, so purchase shoes later in the day, and wear the thickest sock you'd normally wear.
- *Wear low heels.* Keep heels below two-and-a-quarter inches, for better balance and stability.
- *Replace soft insoles with more supportive insoles.*[6] Outdoor recreation stores and finer shoe stores offer a variety of inexpensive orthotic insoles that will provide better support for your foot, improve your posture, and increase the comfort of your current footwear. Superfeet® are designed by a podiatrist and, like fine footwear, are fit to the user's foot and activities. Some styles slip into dress shoes, including those with open toes, while others may be cut to fit, replacing your current insole in casual and athletic wear. Custom insoles are also available for

hard-to-fit feet and hard-core athletes. Contact Superfeet for more information or a sales location near you (see Resources).

316. File down or round off the front tip of your shoe, if you trip on the end of your shoe when you walk.

317. TravelSox®7 stimulate blood flow. If you have poor circulation in your legs, your feet get cold, or your legs tend to hurt or swell at the end of the day, TravelSox® may help. Using a patented gradual compression design and Coolmax® fabric, these comfortable socks help stimulate blood flow and reduce swelling in your legs and feet. They have 300 percent more elasticity than similar legwear and a "dress sock" look that will allow you to keep your legs comfortable, energized, and your feet dry at work or play. You will find these and similar products at travel shops.

318. Eliminate traditional shoelaces with Zackaroos™.8 If you have arthritis in your hands and are having difficulty tying your shoes, you might find Zackaroos™ elastic shoe fasteners helpful. These adjustable elastic fasteners insert into the eyelets of your shoes, creating the look of laces, yet, once inserted, allow you to slip your shoe on and off without needing to tie or untie laces. Each package comes in your choice of black or white, with ten elastic straps—enough for one pair of shoes. Children love the variety of beads available for decorating the elastic laces. Look for them in shoe stores.

319. Slip socks and stockings on easily with stocking aid.9 If you have limited reaching ability; pain in your hips, knees, back; or if the act of stretching footwear to go over your foot is painful, try putting your socks or stockings on with an easy-to-use sock or stocking aid. This device works a little like a shoe horn: slip your sock over the flexible, terrycloth-covered base, and it spreads the sock open, making a generous opening for your foot to enter. Slip your foot into the opening, grasp the two attached straps, and gently pull the sock or stocking over your foot.

320. **Sprinkle cornstarch into your nylon stockings** or onto the bottom of your feet and heels, to make it easier to pull stockings on.

321. **Try men's footwear if you wear an ankle or foot orthotic (AFO).** Men's shoes are wider, provide more support, and are often cheaper than women's. As a general rule, a men's style two sizes smaller than your normal women's size will be about the same size.

322. **If you wear two different-sized shoes due to an ankle foot orthotic (AFO) or leg brace:**
    • *Ask your local shoe store if they sell split sizes.*[10] If not, ask if they can order them from a non-retail company like P.W. Miner.
    • *Some retail stores have policies that allow you to purchase shoes in different sizes* without the cost of two pairs. Companies that have "split-size" shoe policies include Nordstrom's department store (the original Mrs. Nordstrom had polio and needed split-size shoes) and Birkenstock. Of course, retailers may vary in their policies, but it pays to ask.
    • *Try the National Odd Shoe Exchange*, a nonprofit organization that deals in donated shoes.
    • *Try Mix Match Shoes*, a company that sells shoes one at a time.

323. **Wear a plastic bag inside your boots.** Boots will slip on and off easier if you slip your foot into a plastic bag first.

Accessories

324. **Use a revolving tie rack to organize necklaces.** They hang tangle free, are easy to select and retrieve, and can be dusted with a feather duster.

325. **Organize small earrings in stacking ice cube trays.** For easier access, you can attach clip-on earrings to a cake cooling rack that is hung on a wall.

326. **Have a jeweler adapt your necklaces and bracelets with toggle clasps.** If fastening tiny hooks and clasps on your jewelry is difficult, add a toggle clasp that has a large circle on one end of the chain and a thin bar on the other end. To fasten, you simply slide the bar end through the circle.

327. **Magna Magic™ Magnetic Clasp Converters[11] are an inexpensive alternative to hard-to-fasten jewelry clasps.** No restringing is necessary; simply attach your jewelry's clasp and jump ring to the magnetic clasp and you're done—putting on your jewelry is a snap. Available in gold-tone or silver-plated at most hobby and jewelry stores.

328. **Eyeglass necklaces[12] keep glasses within easy reach.** Eyeglass necklaces fashionably hold your reading or sunglasses around your neck, without attaching anything to your glasses. Found in beaded or silver- and gold-toned styles, these necklaces end in an attractive O-ring, which looks nice on its own and serves double duty to hold your glasses by just slipping one of the earpieces through the O-ring. Eyeglass necklaces are available at jewelry and outdoor recreation stores.

RESOURCES

Grooming Aids

1. **Long-handled Scissors**
   Aids for Arthritis
   35 Wakefield Drive
   Medford, NJ 08055
   800-654-0707
   www.AidsForArthritis.com.

2. **Pro-Styling Stand**
   Active Forever
   10799 N. 90th Street
   Scottsdale, AZ 85260
   800-377-8033
   www.ActiveForever.com

Clothing and Accessories

3. **Bra-strap Cushions**
   Aids for Arthritis
   35 Wakefield Drive
   Medford, NJ 08055
   800-654-0707
   www.AidsForArthritis.com

4. **Pre-knotted Zipper Ties**
   Silvert's Head Office
   3280 Steeles Avenue West, Suite 18
   Concord, ONT, Canada L4K 2Y2
   800-387-7088
   www.Silverts.com

Footwear

5. **Supportive Footwear**
   www.Merrelboot.com
   www.Keenfootwear.com
   www.Chacousa.com

6. **Superfeet Insoles**
   Superfeet Worldwide, Inc.
   1419 Whitehorn Street
   Ferndale, WA 98248
   800-634-6618
   www.Superfeet.com

7. **TravelSox**
   The Summit South, Suite 450S

300 Centerville Road
Warwick, RI 02886
866-387-6762
wwwTravelSox.com

8. **Zackaroos**
Steven Enterprises
6053 Third Avenue South
Minneapolis, MN 55419
612-869-9794
www.Zackaroos.com

9. **Sock Dressing Aid**
Aids for Arthritis
35 Wakefield Drive
Medford, NJ 08055
800-654-0707
www.AidsForArthritis.com

10. **Split-size Shoes**
National Odd Shoe Exchange
P.O. Box 1120
Chandler, AZ 85244-1120
480-892-3484
www.OddShoe.org

Nordstrom's
888-282-6060
www.Nordstrom.com

Birkenstock
800-451-1459
www.BirkenstockExpress.com

Mix Match Shoes
236 East Knight Street
Eaton Rapids, MI 48827
888-726-9420
www.MixMatchShoes.com

Jewelry and Accessories

11. Magnetic Jewelry Clasps
MagnaJewelry
1924 Elmwood Avenue
Warwick, RI 02888
www.MagnaJewelry.com

12. Eyeglass Necklaces
Chisco Products
2424 South 2570 West
Salt Lake City, UT 84119
800-825-4555
www.chisco.com

CHAPTER 7

Taking Care of You

Arthritis and related conditions can affect your life in so many ways. It might be morning stiffness that dissipates with a hot shower and a couple of pills, or it may be a painful and disabling restriction of movement for even simple everyday activities. Some days it's easy to cope with the challenges; other days it feels as if it would be easier to just give up and admit defeat.

Staying active and involved is possible with a little effort and determination. Begin by identifying your limitations. Look for ways to work around your pain and limitations. Learning how to take care of myself has been an evolutionary process that has taken many years, and continues to this day. With time and a little experimentation, you will find what works best for you.

People living with arthritis may also experience frustrating problems with concentration, memory, information processing, and communication. If you think any of these thought processes have been affected in you or someone you care about, seek help. Discuss your concerns with your doctor.

These stress-relieving leisure tips and activities, will help you take care of you so you will feel more confident and relaxed while managing all the details of your life.

Staying in Touch

Writing

Reduce the writing you must do with these handy tips:

329. Use a computerized or stamped image of your signature. You can create a computerized image of your signature with a scanner (or at a print shop) and use your home computer to electronically sign correspondence and other documents. If you don't have a computer, purchase a signature stamp from your financial institution or office supply store. Check with your bank to see if the signature stamp can be used on your checks as well as on other documents.

330. Purchase a self-inking return-address stamp or preprinted, self-stick labels to use when paying bills, sending cards, or completing forms. Stamps can be ordered in a variety of font styles from office-supply stores or print shops; labels can be printed by your home computer or ordered from a variety of sources. Use whichever works best for you to affix your return address on envelopes and to fill in the name/address sections of documents. Carry a few labels with you so you are prepared when you are asked to fill in your name and address.

331. Use ball point pens. They glide more easily on paper than felt-tip pens or pencils. If gripping a pen is difficult, look for Y-shaped pens, like the PenAgain™,[1] that fits comfortably in the center of your palm, using the natural weight of your hand to push the pen on the paper, or the ergonomically designed Yoropen (pencil, too) that has an offset tip that lets you write in almost any position with less pressure, finger slipping, or other discomfort. Ask about ergonomic pens and pencils at your local office supply store.

332. Use a rubber grip.[2] If holding a pen or pencil is difficult, twist a rubber band around your pen or pencil several times, positioning the rubber band just below the spot where your fingers rest. If you need a more substantial or smoother grip, purchase a small rubber grip from school or office supply stores. The grips come in a variety of shapes and sizes and have a hole in the center; simply push them into position on your pens or pencils.

333. If check writing is difficult due to a lack of fine motor control, try these suggestions:
- *Make a check template* [3] by cutting spaces out of thin cardboard or other material to match the lines on your checks. To use, place the template on top of the check and use the openings as guides for writing. You can also purchase precut templates for notebook paper, stationery, cards and envelopes, as well as one for personal checks, to keep your handwriting in line and more legible.
- *Pay your bills online*, if you have a computer, let your financial institution "write" the checks for you. Ask about this service and any related fees where you bank.
- *Use a debit card* and skip writing of the check altogether (be sure to keep track of your expenditures).

Telephones, Cell Phones, and Voice Mail

334. Keep important and frequently used phone numbers handy. Avoid having to use a heavy phone book by keeping frequently used phone numbers handy on a printed list near each telephone. Using large print to make the names easier to read, list the phone numbers for individuals you call frequently on one page and the numbers of frequently called businesses, doctors, and others (as well as the poison control center and emergency numbers) on another. Make copies of both lists, place them back-to-back, and slip them into clear acetate sheets. Put one list near each phone in your house. If you have a cell phone, enter frequently used numbers into the cell phone directory and use it to look up and dial numbers.

335. **Let your answering machine or voice mail "take your calls."** If it is hard for you to write down contact information, let your answering machine or voice mail take a message. When you are tired or busy, consider screening your calls with caller ID and answer only those that are important to you.

336. **Keep a solar calculator near the phone**, and use it to quickly "write down" the telephone numbers of people who request a call back.

337. **Cut large, heavy telephone directories in half.** If handling a heavy telephone directory is hard on your hands, try dividing large telephone directories into two sections—the yellow pages and the white pages. Use clear tape to add a cardboard cover to the cut ends.
    - *Contact your telephone company to see if you qualify for free of charge, directory-assistance services.* Your doctor will need to document exactly how your disability prevents you from using a telephone book to obtain addresses and phone numbers.
    - *Ask the reference librarian at your local library to find phone numbers,* if you are having a difficult day and do not qualify for directory assistance.
    - *Use the Internet yellow and white pages to look up addresses* and phone numbers anytime day or night.

338. **If dialing a standard telephone is a pain:**
    - *Purchase a large-keypad telephone* and use the palm of your hand to press the buttons. You can purchase these phones from electronics, office, or discount stores. You may want to contact your telephone company's special-needs department regarding telephones with disability-friendly features and accessibility services they may offer.
    - *Look for a phone with an automatic dial feature.* These phones dial your most frequently called

numbers with the touch of just one button; some are even voice operated.

- *Use a speaker phone* to make using the telephone easier. Speaker phones allow you to talk from up to 15 feet away without having to hold the receiver. Speaker phones are available wherever traditional phones are sold.

- *Use your telephone as an intercom system.* Ask your telephone company if "revertive calling" is available in your area. If so, signal and speak to family members in other rooms by simply dialing your telephone number, waiting for a busy signal, and hanging up the receiver; all the phones in your house will ring and individuals can pick up the handsets and speak to each other without hearing a dial tone in the background.

339. **Call, don't write.** If the pain in your hands makes it hard for you to write, reach out and call someone. Most people love to hear from a friend or loved one, and a personal call can communicate so much more than a letter. If concerned about long-distance charges, many cell phone plans provide free calling at night and on weekends or sign up for a VoIP (Voice over Internet Protocol) service and make free calls from your computer. Cable services offer monthly flat-rate long distance calling; you can also purchase low-cost (pennies a minute) calling cards at many retail outlets. For best success, be sure to purchase a phone card from a trusted company like Verizon or AT&T, rather than the cheapest you can find.

340. **Carry a cell phone for safety.** A cell phone goes where you go, so that you can call for help or keep in touch in case of emergency. Often, cell phones work when land lines are down, and service is restored sooner when a natural disaster strikes. Senior/Call Home plans start at as little as $10 a month. For a comparison of mobile phone plans in your area, go to www.LetsTalk.com.

341. Sign up with the Do Not Call Registry[4] to eliminate unnecessary calls. If you want to keep your telephone, including cell phone, number(s) out of the hands of telemarketers, register your phone number with the national Do Not Call Registry. You must register your numbers every two years or your number will be automatically deleted for at least three months. You can register more often however, so pick an annual date (birthday, anniversary, holiday, or beginning or end of the year) to help you remember to keep your numbers registered.

Computers and Technology

342. Embrace ergonomics. Using the computer can be hard on the joints in your fingers, hands, arms, neck, and back. If you use one regularly, it is important to investigate the ergonomically designed products that will make working at your computer most comfortable for you. Visit a full-service computer store to learn about and test drive ergonomic keyboards, mice, pens, and other devices.

343. Keep in touch electronically. If you have access to a computer, e-mail to family and friends. Typing your message is often easier than gripping a pen and writing one; as a bonus, your message gets there faster and without the need of paper, stamps, or envelopes. If you do not have Internet service at home, senior centers and libraries offer access to the Internet, and staff can help you set up a free e-mail account on any number of free servers (Yahoo, Google, Hotmail, etc.). Call your librarian to arrange a time for her to show you how to set up and use an e-mail account. If you have specific concerns about how computer usage may affect you, contact a physical or occupational therapist for an evaluation and suggestions.

344. Find the right keyboard. A number of keyboards on the market are designed to eliminate the back, shoulder, neck, hand, and wrist pain of using a computer. Try an ergonomic or soft-touch keyboard at your favorite computer store, or ask if you can try one at home for a few days before you purchase it.

345. Eliminate wrist strain with an ergonomically designed mouse. Numerous devices are designed to eliminate the hand pain that can come with computer work. In addition to an ergonomically designed mouse, available in right- and left-hand styles, vertical mice, track balls, pens, and other designs are also available. Ask to try different styles at your local computer or office supply store before you buy. Look for devices with a raised, soft, cushioned gel pad to support the wrist.

346. Use a notebook (laptop) computer. Notebook computers are smaller, lightweight, and portable, allowing you to work in a position that is most comfortable for you, even if that changes frequently. Newer computers even come with touch-screen technology built in, so you do not have to make as many keystrokes or mouse movements. Find your most comfortable position on a desk, table, or in your lap, or work on an adjustable surface like a drafting table or ironing board. If you choose to work with the computer in your lap, be sure to use a lapboard or notebook desk, a stable platform to set your computer on so it does not overheat and burn your legs. Some platforms are raised, and you can adjust the angle of the platform to give you even more comfort options.

347. Use the accessibility features on your computer. If sore joints in your fingers and hands, or tremors, make it difficult to type, the accessibility features built into your computer can make life easier. Check your computer help files for information on accessibility options and learn how to adjust the speed of mouse clicks, key strokes, and the pointer; increase the size of the font or the color contrast of the display; and activate warning sounds to make your computer easier to use. For people with the use of only one hand, sticky keys allow you to press one key after the other (Ctrl/Alt/Delete) to respond as if you pressed them at the same time.

348. **Improve your posture**, by using a large font (18- to 24-point) when creating or reading a document on the computer. This will help you sit up straighter, reducing pain and helping you read your document more easily.

349. **Plug all your computer equipment into one power-strip surge protector**, so that you can press one switch to turn all the equipment on or off at one time.

350. **Use a PDA to keep you organized.** An electronic pocket organizer or PDA, like a Palm Pilot or Blackberry, will keep your address book, appointment calendar, important phone numbers, notes, and to-do lists all in one place; some include voice recognition or a built-in tape recorder to make recording information easier. You might consider one with a mobile phone component, so you only have one electronic device to keep track of. Before you buy, try these devices out at your local computer or electronics store to see which features are best for you. Evaluate any or all of the following:
   • Weight and size
   • Screen display size and brightness controls
   • Button size and pressure needed to input data
   • Clarity of sound
   • Ease of use and learning curve
   • Ease of backing up information and synchronizing to your computer
   • Ability and ease of consolidating or combining data within the device (i.e. business card names into your address book)
   • Technical support

- Repair record
- Helpful software

351. Program your computer to avoid repetitive stress injuries. Working on a computer can be very hard on the joints, especially the neck, shoulders, and hands. Program your computer to remind you to take breaks regularly. Software programs[5] are available that will remind you to take a break and provide you with helpful exercises to avoid joint injury.

352. Speak instead of type, using voice-recognition software.[6] If your joints are really sore, and writing and typing have become a chore, or you simply want to reduce the wear and tear of typing, voice-recognition software, like Dragon Naturally Speaking, can open new doors of communication. Once you train the program to recognize your speech, you can speak into a microphone, and the computer will type your words with up to 99% accuracy—faster than you could type them. You can also send e-mail, instant messages, and surf the web just by speaking into a microphone.

353. Add pictures to voice calls. VoIP is an emerging technology that allows you to make free calls through your computer. Another advantage of VoIP services (such as Skype) is that VoIP not only transmits voice communication but, with the addition of a simple and inexpensive camera that connects to your computer, you can also see the person you are talking with. This is a great way to connect with loved ones anywhere in the world and watch grandchildren grow.

Keeping the Fun in Your Life

Reading

354. Take advantage of the library's collection of large-print and audio books that you can listen to or read from your lap. If you have trouble holding a book for any length of time, the *Large-Type Books in Print* directory has thousands of entries, including books and periodicals, published in large print. This reference book is available at most major libraries.

355. **Read books on your computer.** BookShare.org scans books and makes them available to people with disabilities, including visual impairments, learning disabilities, and mobility impairments, that affect the ability to read, hold a book, or turn a page. For more information, go to www.BookShare.org.

356. **Search and reserve books online.** Save yourself a trip to the library—search and reserve books online using the library's Internet connection. When your books are ready to be picked up, the library will let you know; some communities have volunteers who will drop off and pick up library books at your door at no charge. Ask for information and assistance from your local librarian.

357. **Call the library reference department for assistance.** If you want to know a fact or figure, contact information for a local support group, how to spell a word, or even the name and phone number of a local restaurant, the reference librarian may be able to assist you. They have many resources at their fingertips, including the ability to do an Internet search for you.

358. **Use an eraser to help turn pages.** If your fingers give you trouble turning the pages in a book or magazine, use the eraser end of a pencil, a rubber finger, or tacky solution on your finger to help you turn pages. Tacky solutions and rubber fingers can be found where office supplies are sold.

Watching Television

359. **Use a universal remote control.**[7] In a few simple steps, a universal remote can be programmed to operate all

of your TVs, DVD/VCRs, stereos, and other electronic equipment, saving you time and the clutter of multiple remotes on your coffee table. Tek Partner makes a Giant Universal Remote Control with illuminated buttons—three times the size of conventional remotes. This remote control is easy to hold, it's easy to find the right button, and it can replace up to four standard remotes, operating any combination of TVs, VCRs, and cable boxes. For ordering information, see the Resources section.

360. **Keep your remote from getting lost** by attaching a piece of hook-and-loop fastener tape (like Velcro™) to the remote and the side of the TV, chair, or table. You might do the same with your phone or cell phone in your car or any other place they might tend to get lost.

361. **Join a video subscription service.** If visiting the video store and sorting through movies is hard for you, or you tend to forget those video rentals on top of the TV and late charges pile up, sign up for a subscription service that offers unlimited rentals that you can keep as long as you want. Netflix (www.NetFlix.com) has a number of plans; DVDs are mailed to your door, along with a prepaid mailer to return watched movies. Blockbuster and Wal-Mart also offer monthly rates.

Playing Games

362. **Play games.** Just as physical activity keeps your body strong, mental activity keeps your mind sharp and agile and keeps you from concentrating on your pain and discomfort. Challenge yourself with word games and puzzles, read, stay informed about the world around you, and try new things.

363. **Adapt game board pieces for easier handling.** If you have trouble handling game pieces, try substituting

larger items like Lego® blocks, empty plastic pill bottles, chess pieces, or little plastic finger puppets. To adapt cardboard game pieces that are too thin and unstable to pick up or set down easily, glue an extra piece of cardboard on the bottom to make the base slightly larger.

364. **Place game boards on a lazy-susan.** If you have arthritis, a revolving game board may make it easier to join in the fun. Purchase a lazy-Susan turntable from a kitchen department or cabinet shop and place the game board on top; the board can easily be turned to meet each player's reach. If the game board is still too far for a comfortable reach, place an easy-to-grasp-and-slide placemat, cookie sheet, or cutting board under the turntable and slide it closer when it's time to make your move.

365. **Buy deluxe versions of games that use all the senses to aid play.** For example, the Scrabble Deluxe Edition[8] has ridges that hold the tiles in place and a board that rotates to face the person playing the new word. Tactile overlays may be added to the tiles and board, which helps in grasping and placing pieces, especially for those with visual or fine motor impairments. You will also find large-sized playing cards, card holders, card shufflers, and games like bingo, Chinese checkers, Tic Tac Toe, Uno, dominoes, chess, and checkers for people with special needs.

Crafts and Needlework

If you love to knit or crochet, sew, or be crafty but find standard methods and tools too hard to use, don't give up on your favorite pastime, just change your tools and techniques.

366. **Use bamboo, soft touch, circular, and lighted knitting needles and crochet hooks.** Bamboo hooks and needles

are lightweight, and their natural surface holds the yarn just enough to keep stitches even. Circular needles help to support some of the weight of your project. Wrap a rubber band around the handle of your crochet hooks, or purchase flexible, flattened square crochet hooks or Soft Touch hooks that are ergonomically designed to be easier to hold and eliminate stress on the hands and joints. If you find yourself straining to see what you are working on, hooks and needles with lighted ends may ease the strain on your eyes. Also, try working with wool or wool blend yarns, which are more elastic and forgiving that cotton and synthetic fibers. Specialty hooks and needles are available at fine craft shops.[9]

367. **Use an embroidery hoop with clamps.** Put your embroidery or needlepoint work in the hoop, attach it to a table or chair, and it greatly reduces the stress on your hands. Try leather or rubber fingertip thimbles to loosen your grip on the needle. Also, try working on a broader linen weave that is easier to both see and push the needle through.

368. **Place your portable sewing machine on an adjustable ironing board.** This will allow you to adjust the height of the machine for maximum comfort. An adjustable ironing board can be a wonderful work surface for many projects.

369. **Avoid bending to pick up pins.** A magnetized screw-driver, reacher, or yardstick with a magnet glued to the bottom will pick up steel straight pins and other metal objects without bending.

370. **Sewing and mending are easier if you use lightweight electric scissors** and either straight pins with large balls on top or glass-headed quilting pins.

371. **Use a hanging magnifying glass.** To help you see what you are working on, without getting a crick in your

neck, try wearing a magnifying glass specially designed to hang around your neck. Find these unique products at sewing or craft stores.

372. **Use a potato to thread needles.** To make it easier to thread a needle, stick the needle into an apple or a potato and place it on a shelf or counter that's at eye level. Then, you can easily see to thread the eye. Or, you might purchase self-threading needles. Rethread needles as soon as the thread is used up so your needles are always ready to use. Self-threading needles are available at fabric stores.

Houseplants

373. **Monitor houseplant moisture from afar with moisture monitoring sticks.** If it's painful to reach up to determine when houseplants need to be watered, invest in moisture monitoring "sticks" that change appearance and let you know at a glance when your plants need water. Numerous decorative and whimsical styles are available at garden centers.

374. **Mist plants with a personal mister.** If squeezing the trigger of a traditional plant mister is hard on your joints, try using a personal mister designed to cool you on hot summer days. Simply fill the easy-to-grasp bottle, turn the thumb screw, and the mister will spray a fine mist over your plants until you turn it off again. The Misty Mate[10] comes in 12- and 24-ounce models. For extra humidity in the winter, locate plants near a humidifier.

375. **Replace heavy watering cans with a lightweight indoor plant hose.** If lifting and carrying a heavy watering can makes watering houseplants a pain, consider purchasing an indoor plant hose from your local garden-supply center. Attach the lightweight and easy-to-manage hose to a kitchen or other faucet, and you'll

likely be able to reach all the plants in your house. You might also use a plastic sports drink bottle with a flexible straw to water hard-to-reach plants; squeeze the bottle and the water runs out of the straw and into the container.

376. **Wear gloves or old socks to dust plants.** To dust the leaves on indoor plants, wear a pair of cotton gloves (or old socks) and dampen them with warm water. With one hand on top and one on the bottom, use both hands to wipe off the leaves. This works well with furniture too; just use a little lemon oil or furniture polish.

Exercise

377. **Use it or lose it.** Recent studies show that mild to moderate exercise reduces pain and enhances your overall well-being. Check with your local physical or occupational therapist, hospital, healthcare clinic, or health maintenance organization (HMO) for suggestions on exercises that are best for your individual situation.

378. **Stay limber and reduce pain by walking and stretching.** Simple stretching exercises can be done in bed or under the moist heat of a hot shower. Walking will loosen up painful muscles, get your heart moving, and free your mind of hurtful thoughts. Getting out of the house and doing something good for your body will bring lasting rewards.

379. **Try Pilates, yoga, or tai chi.** Exercise does not have to be hard on your joints. Core-strengthening modalities like Pilates, yoga, or tai chi gently stretch and strengthen your body, reducing pain and stiffness along the way. Ask your local hospital, healthcare clinic, or HMO about low-cost classes, or consult class offerings at your local health and fitness club.

380. Swim in a warm pool. Water helps to support your body so that any exercise you do is less stressful on painful joints. Water offers the added advantage of providing more resistance than air, so everything you do has added benefit. Look for a "warm-water pool"; the higher temperature of the water is more soothing than that of a regular pool.

Restaurants and Entertainment

381. Call ahead to check accessibility. If you have difficulty walking very far, or if you use a walker or wheelchair, call ahead to restaurants, theaters, and other venues before you leave home, to ask if they are accessible. Ask about parking facilities, where the restrooms are located, the most convenient entrance, and so on.

382. Choose quieter places to spend your time out. Noisy environments can add undue stress and deplete you of energy. Look for restaurants with drapes, low ceilings, and carpeted or vinyl floors. Avoid establishments with wooden floors, loud music, multiple TVs, or high unfinished ceilings. As a safeguard, carry earplugs in your purse or pocket.

383. Choose well-lit restaurants. Restaurants with dim or subdued lighting make it difficult to walk across the room, read the menu, or even communicate with dinner companions.

384. Purchase tickets and gift certificates online. Use your phone to purchase tickets to plays, concerts, and movies; dinner reservations; or gift certificates to restaurants. Charge to a credit or debit card and have the certificates or tickets mailed to your home. While online, check out seating and menus.

RESOURCES

Writing Aids

1. **Ergonomic Pens and Pencils**
   Pacific Writing Instruments
   650-355-2640
   www.PenAgain.com.

   Yoropen Corporation
   www.YoropenCorp.com

2. **Pen and Pencil Grips**

3. **Writing Templates**
   Abilitations
   P.O. Box 922668
   Norcross, GA 30010-2668
   800-850-8602
   www.abilitations.com

Telephone Aids

4. **Do Not Call Registry**
   888-382-1222
   www.DoNotCall.gov

Computer Use

5. **Repetitive Stress-prevention Software**
   Remedy Interactive, Inc.
   480 Gate Five Road, Suite 130
   Sausalito, CA 94965
   800-776-5545
   www.RSIguard.com

6. **Speech Recognition Software**
   Nuance
   1 Wayside Road
   Burlington, MA 01803
   781-565-5000
   www.Nuance.com/NaturallySpeaking

Entertainment and Games

7. Giant Remote Control
Active Forever
10799 North 90th Street
Scottsdale, AZ 85260
800-377-8033
www.ActiveForever.com

8. Deluxe and Adaptive Games
Independent Living Aids, Inc.
200 Robbins Lane
Jericho, NY 11753
800-537-2118
www.IndependentLiving.com

S&S® Worldwide
P.O. Box 513
75 Mill Street
Colchester, CT 06415
1-800-288-9941
www.ssww.com

Hobbies and Crafts

9. Knitting and Crocheting Supplies
Clover Needlecraft, Inc.
13438 Alondra Boulevard
Cerritos, California 90703-2315
800-233-1703
www.clover-USA.com

10. Personal Misters
Misty Mate, Inc.
955 North Fiesta Boulevard, Suite 1
Gilbert, AZ 85233
800-233-6478
www.MistyMate.com

CHAPTER 8

Getting Out and About

Life is busy! Sometimes it seems that errands and outings are taking up more and more time. Planning ahead and being more organized will help you increase your efficiency and reduce the wear and tear on your body.

Before you leave home, take a moment to look over your planned stops. Is it a good time of day to be going to the library or post office? Will the drive-up windows at the bank be open? Are you positive the prescriptions are ready at the pharmacy?

Rearrange the order of your stops to make errands most convenient for you. If you're prone to forgetting the sequence, write it down. Leave low-priority stops at the bottom of the list, so if you get tired you can leave them for another time.

Sometimes your diagnosis and/or medications can impact your perception, reaction time, and your ability to drive safely. Be realistic about your abilities. Have someone else drive you if necessary. Discuss with a doctor your concerns about driving and see it adjusting your medications or the time you take them can improve your ability to drive.

With a realistic itinerary and a dash of creativity, you can still get out and do many of the things you want to do.

Around Town

Shopping

385. Push a grocery cart for added stability when walking.
Some department stores have carts for patrons to use
and a growing number of stores and shopping malls
provide three-wheeled battery-operated scooters for
shoppers who tire easily or have trouble walking. Scooters are usually available on a first-come, first-served
basis at the service desk or information booth. Use the
scooter and save your energy for more important things.

386. Shop online or by mail to save time and energy. In a
notebook or the memo area of your personal checkbook
keep a record of all mail-order or online company information. You'll have a complete record of the purchase
should you need to contact the company for any reason.

387. Shop early. In your wallet or purse, keep a list of people
you need to buy gifts for, including sizes, and favorite
brands or colors. When you are out and you encounter
a sale, consult your gift list and purchase items
throughout the year, avoiding last-minute gift shopping
or hectic holiday times.

388. Wrap holiday gifts as soon as you purchase them, so
that you won't have to fuss with them as the days
become more hectic. Wrapping a few at a time is easier
on the hands than doing the whole bunch at once. If you
must wrap many gifts at one time, use an adjustable
ironing board as a table; you can raise or lower the board
easily and sit or stand to suit your needs. Wrap packages in different colors for different recipients and you
will know at a glance which gifts are for whom.

Errands

389. File an absentee ballot to avoid leaving home to vote.
Contact the city clerk in your area for a permanent

absentee ballot. You will receive a ballot several weeks before each election, and then cast your vote by mail.

390. Do your banking from home:
- *Bank by mail.* Ask the bank for stamped, self-addressed envelopes for mailing deposits and payments. Have the bank process your transactions and return the receipts to you or track them online. If possible, arrange for your checks to be automatically deposited to your account.
- *Ask about bill-paying assistance.* Some banks will send a representative to your home to help you with your bill paying and record keeping.
- *Pay household bills electronically.* Set up payments once and each month, utility, credit card, and other bill payments will be automatically deducted from your account. You'll receive documentation of the transactions.
- *Bank online*, where you can check deposits, authorize payments, and track all activity on your account any time, day or night. With a few clicks of a mouse, your bills are paid and the bank does the rest. Shop around and choose a bank that offers the services you need at little or no cost to you.

391. Plan a convenient route to make shopping and errands easier. Think over the route for the stops on your errand trips and write it down. Before you leave home, consider: Is this a good time of day to be going to the library or post office? Will the drive-up windows at the bank be open? Will there be lines? Arrange the sequence of stops in an order that is most convenient for you. If a sequence of four or five errands is too tiring, make trips with fewer stops; do one or two errands at a time and then go home, get organized for the next set of errands, and go again when you feel rested.

Car and Driving

Making Your Vehicle More Accessible

392. Use a seatbelt extender handle[1] to avoid over reaching and pain. If reaching over your shoulder is painful on hands, arms, or shoulders, an Easy Reach seatbelt handle can extend your reach and make pulling the seat belt easier. The 12-inch rubber extension handle simply snaps over your current seatbelt. Available in beige, black, white and one that glows in the dark for nighttime driving. Ask about them in automotive departments.

393. Install handles to help you get in and out of your car. The CarCaddie™ is a portable handle that straps around the top of the window frame, providing a cushion grip for easing yourself in and out of the car. The buckle is ergonomically designed to make it easy to open and close. Because it is adjustable and not permanently installed, it can be moved to other vehicles, although it is not suitable for convertibles or other vehicles without an enclosed window frame.

   A similar accessory, the Handybar™,[2] is a super-strong, removable, personal support bar handle that inserts into a U-shaped plate installed on your vehicle door frame, for both driver and passenger side doors. Constructed of a forged steel shaft with a soft non-slip grip handle, it will safely support up to 350 pounds.

394. Use a beaded seat cover, to make it easier to get into or out of your car. The beads not only make sliding into your seat easier, they make long drives more comfortable and protect you from seats that are too hot in the summer and too cold in the winter.

395. Use a transfer disc to get in and out of your car. The Flexi-Disc[3] works like a lazy-Susan for people. Made of tough durable fabric, this flexible disc allows you to turn your body into place without twisting, giving a better sense of stability and security when getting into or out of a vehicle. Simply place the disc on the car seat and use the swivel action to turn into place. The fabric conforms to the user and folds for easy storage between uses. The disk can also assist in getting in and out of a bed or chair.

396. Install an automatic car starter/keyless entry system.[4] If you have difficulty using keys, an automatic car starter with keyless entry system might be helpful. Install one on any automatic transmission, fuel-injection vehicle, and you can lock, unlock, or start your car from up to 2,500 feet away.

397. Install turning automotive seating,[5] if you use a wheelchair or scooter in your vehicle. The seat, which comes in several models, some utilizing or matching existing seating, can be installed in many types and brands of vehicles, including sedans, SUVs, wagons, crossovers, minivans, pickup trucks, and full-size vans. Hand controls allow you to pivot and lower the seat to your level, making transferring easier. A companion lift can pick up your wheelchair and load it in and out of your vehicle; one model even converts into a wheelchair, making the lift unnecessary. Check with your dealer about compatibility with your auto, van, or truck.

398. Use a gas cap wrench.[6] If opening a gas cap is hard because of weak hands or sore muscles, there is an easier way. The Gas Cap Wrench has a long handle and a formed X shape, designed to fit over bar style gas caps and give you extra leverage to twist and turn the cap with ease. Look for this or similar products at an automotive store.

Traveling by Car

For helpful driving tips, check with your local Department of Transportation or AAA office or visit the National Highway

Transportation Safety Administration (NHTSA) website at
www.safercar.gov.

399. **Keep two hands safely on the wheel.** You know you
should keep two hands on the steering wheel to safely
negotiate emergencies, but safe placement of your
hands has changed with the addition of airbags. To
keep your hands (with rings, sharp fingernails, etc.)
from hindering air bag deployment and possibly doing
serious damage to your face, the recommended driving
position is at nine and three o'clock on the outside of
the wheel (usually where manufacturers place a hand
grip). Safe travels!

400. **Pack a small overnight bag with emergency supplies.** In a zipper-locked plastic bag, pack medications, mints, gum, high-protein snacks (nuts, energy
bars), candy, a pack of cards, a book, and a change of
clothes. Keep it within easy reach while driving, and
if you need a snack along the way or you are delayed
in your travels, you and your passengers will have
what you need.

401. **Keep a safety kit in the car for emergencies.** Be prepared for whatever the season may bring by keeping a
box of "necessities" in the trunk of your car. For example: water bottles, rain gear, sunglasses, and extra socks
for spring/summer; extra sweaters, hats, scarves, mittens and gloves, and a blanket for winter. Also, fill three
or four empty coffee cans (wide-mouth plastic containers may also work) with sand or kitty litter for extra
traction when you need it. Put a bright strip of reflector
tape around the cans and they can double as safety
cones; if you get stuck or break down, put them around
your car so oncoming traffic will know to slow down.
Put candles and waterproof matches in one or two of
the cans (fill these cans only half full of sand); if you get
stuck in the cold, the candle can add just enough heat to

keep you comfortable while you wait for help. (Be sure to crack the window for ventilation.)

402. Use old bedsheets to protect your upholstery. When transporting children to and from after-school sporting activities you might want to carry a few old sheets to protect car seats from dirty uniforms.

403. Stay warm when traveling with electric car blanket. For extra warmth when traveling on a cold winter's day, plug a specially designed electric car blanket into your vehicle's power port or cigarette lighter. Look in automotive or discount department stores for a high-quality fleece blanket, large enough for two people, and a power cord long enough to reach the back seat.

404. Try a sheepskin seat belt cover. If you find wearing a seatbelt uncomfortable due to sensitive skin or body pain, a genuine sheepskin cover will cushion the pressure of the belt against your neck and chest and make driving or riding more comfortable. Available in automotive sections.

405. Support your legs and back on long trips. To reduce leg and back pain on long-distance drives or commutes, Drivease™,[7] a simple but effective ergonomic device, can really add to your comfort. Position the firm, flexible support under your right leg to aid circulation and support the sciatic nerve and lower back, helping you to maintain a comfortable driving posture.

406. Use a Sticky Pad to keep accessories within reach. Keep loose change, sunglasses, even your cell phone handy and in place with the Sticky Pad. Just peel away the self-adhesive backing and adhere the pad to a clean, dry dash. (For safety's sake be sure to apply in a spot away from the air bag, as items propelled by the air bag deployment can be very dangerous.) The top side has a tacky surface that will keep small items from sliding around under normal driving conditions. If the pad loses its stick, just wash it to revitalize; it's reusable when applied to soft, vinyl surfaces. You might also find these pads helpful in the kitchen, family room, or bedroom to keep remotes and other small items within reach. Purchase where auto supplies and accessories are sold.

407. **Adjust your mirrors to eliminate blind spots.** If you find turning your head to check that blind spot a pain in the neck, here is a simple tip to reset your side view mirrors and make it possible to check traffic easily without twisting your neck and body:

Sit in your car as if you were driving. To adjust the driver's side mirror, lean toward the driver's side window until the top of your head just touches the glass; adjust the mirror so you can just see the tip of your rear bumper. Then, lean toward the center of the car and do the same with the passenger side mirror. When you sit in the driving position, you should not see your car at all but you will have a clear view of the lane next to you. With your mirrors set this way, as traffic leaves your sight in your rearview mirror, it will pop into your side mirror; when you can no longer see it in the side mirror, your peripheral vision will pick it up. To change lanes, you only need to tip or turn your head slightly to take a peek; no more twisting around to see what is behind you.

408. **Install panoramic and wide angle mirrors to keep from overextending your neck.**
   - *Panoramic rear-view mirror.* Gain a larger view of the road and make it easier and safer to change lanes, merge, and exit highways, without twisting your neck, by clipping a panoramic rear-view mirror over your factory-installed mirror. Look for regular shatterproof, distortion-free, antiglare mirrors in two sizes: regular, to fit automobiles, and large, for vans, trucks, and SUVs.

- *Auxiliary blind-spot mirror.* Attach this to the top of your side-view mirror to give you a wide-angle view, virtually eliminating blind spots. Made of impact-resistant black ABS plastic, it mounts easily above or below your existing mirror with the use of a mini wrench (included) and your screwdriver. Available in two sizes—standard, for automobiles and large, for SUVs, trucks, and vans. (Note: As with your passenger side mirror, objects are closer than they appear.)
- *Driveway mirror.* Get a better view of what's behind you when backing out of your driveway with a large, convex mirror (like you see in banks and stores) that gives you a wide-angle view of blind curves, children playing, and toys. Lightweight and break-resistant, the mirror installs easily with the included mounting bracket. Choose one with a built-in visor to reduce glare from overhead light. For household safety, one may also be mounted to give you a wide-angle view of your entryway from another room or floor.

Specialty mirrors[8] are found in automotive shops or departments or from the online retailers.

409. **Install a back-up alert warning alarm and light.**[9] For added safety when backing up, install a back-up alert light in the tail light of your light truck, RV, car, or van. Whenever your vehicle is in reverse, it automatically emits a continuous beeping sound. Installation is as easy a changing a light bulb.

410. **Install a back-up camera on your vehicle.**[10] Back up with less twisting and more peace of mind by installing a back-up camera. These devices are becoming less expensive and more readily available all the time. A wireless version installs easily, without professional help, on your license plate holder and plugs into your back-up light to transmit the picture to a separate dashboard console. Check out different

models at automotive stores and in the automotive or electronic section of some discount department stores.

411. **Carry a portable jump starter for emergencies.**[11] If you are traveling across country or just across town, keep a portable jump starter (a battery charger for your car) in the trunk. When your car won't start, connect the cables to your battery, and the jump starter gives you enough "juice" to start your car, without another person or vehicle involved. Most automotive departments carry a compact portable jump starter, sometimes with a tire inflator, light, and emergency safety reflectors. Be sure to keep the starter charged.

412. **Jump your car without opening the hood.** If it is hard for you to get out of the car and open the hood, or you get confused or outright scared at the thought of jump-starting your car (now, where do I attach the red wire???) the Easy Quick Jumper[12] is for you. This handy device charges your car through the power ports or cigarette lighters of two vehicles—no need to open the hood or connect cables to the battery. Simply plug one end into the power port/cigarette lighter socket of your car and the other into another car, wait five minutes, and start the engine. LED lights confirm correct connection and charging, so you know you are doing everything correctly; the 18-foot cord makes connection easy even in tight spaces and it's compact enough to fit in the glove compartment. Compare with other models at automotive departments or online.

413. **Don't forget your personal disabled-driver/passenger windshield placard.** Disabled parking permits are honored in most states, including on a rental car or in a car in which you are a passenger. If you forget to bring your permit with you, your only option will be to visit the nearest Motor Vehicle department office and request a temporary permit; don't be surprised if they want to

see a doctor's letter certifying your disability or medical condition. Don't leave home without it!

Weekend Getaways and Extended Travel

Leaving the comforts of home for an extended vacation or a day trip to meet friends, can sometimes present obstacles and challenges, yet it's vitally important to your physical, mental, and emotional health that you stay active and connected to people and places near and far. With a little extra planning and preparation, you can reduce the stress and energy needed to solve problems and inconveniences. These tips will give you a good start.

414. Use a travel club or the Internet to make traveling easier. Do your research and planning online, or let someone else do it for you. Specialized travel agencies are helpful when choosing unfamiliar or foreign destinations, when you have complicated arrangements or restrictions, or mobility and energy concerns. To be prepared for most situations, seek out information in the following areas:
- *Weather*
- *What to pack*
- *Driving*
    Road conditions
    Construction and detours
    Rest stop locations and accessibility
- *Air travel*
    Reservations
    On-plane special needs
        – Seating location and selection
        – Meal options
        – Service animals
        – Wheelchair access
    Security and medically related concerns
    Airport services and assistance

- *Accessibility issues*
    Hotel accommodations and services
    Transportation
    Points of interests
    Restaurants and restroom access

Once your arrangements are complete and you leave for your getaway, accept that obstacles, delays, glitches, and surprises will occur. Chose to accept them in the spirit of adventure. Think of the memories you'll have and the stories you'll be able to tell!

RESOURCES

1. **Seatbelt Extender**
   ElderStore
   6820 Meadowridge Court, Suite A-9
   Alpharetta, GA 30005
   888-833-8875
   www.ElderStore.com

2. **Car Handles**
   Dynamic Living
   95 W. Dudleytown Road
   Bloomfield, CT 06002
   888-940-0605
   www.Dynamic-Living.com

3. **Flexi Disc Transfer Disc**
   Phil-E-Slide, Inc.
   9 Industrial Way
   Atkinson, NH 03811
   866-675-4338
   www.Phil-e-Slide-US.com

4. **Automatic Car Starter/Keyless Entry System**
   GNU Industries, Inc.
   1919 NW 19th Street, Building 1A

Ft. Lauderdale, FL 33311
800-780-1409
www.CommandoAlarms.com

5. **Turning Automotive Seating**
Bruno Independent Living Aids, Inc.
1780 Executive Drive
P.O. Box 84
Oconomowoc, WI 53066
800-882-8183
www.bruno.com

6. **Gas Cap Wrench**
Arthritis Supplies
The Wright Stuff, Inc.
135 Floyd G. Harrell Drive
Grenada, MS 38901
877-750-0376
www.ArthritisSupplies.com

7. **Drivease**
AutoSport Catalog
P.O. Box 9036
Charlottesville, VA 22906
800-953-0814
www.AutoSportCatalog.com

8. **Automotive Mirrors**
Driving Comfort
P.O. Box 9036
Charlottesville, VA 22906
www.DrivingComfort.com

9. **Back-up Alert**
DesignTech International, LLC.
1 Viper Way
Vista, CA 92081
800-876-0800
www.DesignTech-Intl.com

10. Back-up Camera
AJ Prindle
301 Sonoco Drive
Louisiana, MO 63353
800-780-9356
www.AJPrindle.com

11. Portable Jump Starter
Driving Comfort
P.O. Box 9036
Charlottesville, VA 22906
www.DrivingComfort.com

12. Cigarette Lighter Jump Starter
AutoSport Catalog
P.O. Box 9036
Charlottesville, VA 22906
800-953-0814
www.AutoSportCatalog.com

Resources

SUPPORT ORGANIZATIONS

American College of Rheumatology
1800 Century Place, Suite 250
Atlanta, GA 30345-4300
404-633-3777
www.rheumatology.org

Arthritis Foundation
P.O. Box 7669
Atlanta, GA 30357-0669
800-283-7800
www.arthritis.org

National Institute of Arthritis and Musculoskeletal and
Skin Diseases (NIAMS)
Information Clearinghouse
National Institutes of Health
1 AMS Circle
Bethesda, MD 20892-3675
301-495-4484
Toll Free: 877-22-NIAMS (226-4267)
TTY: 301–565–2966
Website: www.niams.nih.gov

National Institutes for Health (NIH)
9000 Rockville Pike
Bethesda, Maryland 20892
301-496-4000
www.health.nih.gov

MedLine Plus
www.MedLinePlus.gov
Online medical information source.

Web MD
www.WebMD.com
Online medical information source.

ACCESSIBILITY AIDS AND PRODUCTS

Abilitations
P.O. Box 922668
Norcross, GA 30010-2668
800-850-8602
www.abilitations.com
Source for adaptable and ergonomic writing aids,
including pen and pencil grips and writing templates.

Active Forever
10799 N. 90th Street
Scottsdale, AZ 85260
800-377-8033
www.ActiveForever.com
Home and activity adaptability aids, including lifting
straps to make carrying loads easier, pro-styling dryer
stand, and giant remote controls.

Aids for Arthritis
35 Wakefield Drive
Medford, NJ 08055
800-654-0707
www.AidsForArthritis.com
Good source for home, personal, and hobby adaptability
and accessibility items, including long-handled scissors,
bra strap cushions, and sock dressing aid.

AJ Prindle
301 Sonoco Drive
Louisiana, MO 63353
800-780-9356
www.AJPrindle.com
Source for everything that makes automotive travel easier
and more comfortable, including back-up camera systems.

AmeriBag Inc.
Consumer Services Department
5 AmeriBag Drive
Kingston, NY 12401
888-758-1636
www.AmeriBag.com
Ergonomic and stylish handbags and luggage.

Arthritis Supplies
The Wright Stuff, Inc.
135 Floyd G. Harrell Drive
Grenada, MS 38901
877-750-0376
www.Mobility-Aids.com
Accessories for canes and walkers and other mobility aids.

Arthritically Correct! Products
P.O. Box 4047
Stateline, NV 89449
408-445-2011
www.ArthriticallyCorrect.com
Home adaptability aids, including the EZ Key.

Assistance Dog United Campaign
1221 Sebastopol Road
Santa Rosa, CA 95407
800 284-DOGS (3647)
www.AssistanceDogUnitedCampaign.org
Information on service dogs.

AutoSport Catalog
P.O. Box 9036
Charlottesville, VA 22906
800-953-0814
www.AutoSportCatalog.com
Source for automotive tools, gadgets, accessories, and
customizing items, including the electric car blanket, the
Drivease lower back/lumbar support device that makes

long car trips more comfortable, and a jump starter that works from the in-dash cigarette lighter.

Baggy Buddy
P.O. Box 4269
Ft. Lauderdale, FL 33338
www.BaggyBuddy.com

B.A. Maze, Inc.
c/o R. Mazur
43311 Joy Road
Canton, MI 48187
800-708-6736
www.PurrfectOpener.com
The source for the PurrfectOpener, a multipurpose can/container opener.

Bed Handles, Inc.
2905 SW 19th Street
Blue Springs, Missouri 64015
800-725-6903
www.BedHandles.com
The name says it all: the source for bed handles to make turning over and transfers easier.

Birkenstock
800-451-1459
www.BirkenstockExpress.com
Source for split-size shoes.

Black & Decker, Inc.
101 Schilling Road
Hunt Valley, MD 21031
800-544-6986
www.BlackandDecker.com
Manufacturer of the Powered Kitchen Scrubber and other helpful household appliances and tools.

Bruno Independent Living Aids, Inc.
1780 Executive Drive
P.O. Box 84
Oconomowoc, WI 53066
800-882-8183
www.Bruno.com
Source for vehicular adaptability/accessibility products,
including lifts and turning automotive seating.

The Cane Mart
www.CaneMart.com
Canes and accessories.

CaseLogic
6303 Dry Creek Parkway
Longmont, CO 80503
888-666-5780
www.CaseLogic.com
Good source of fashionable, adaptable luggage, bags, and
accessories like large-tabbed zipper pulls and the Armrest
Organizer.

Chaco USA
www.Chacousa.com
Fashionable supportive footwear for all lifestyles.

Chef's Planet®
2120 E. Rose Garden, Suite E1
Phoenix, AZ 85024
602-906-3600
www.ChefsPlanet.com

Chisco Products
2424 South 2570 West
Salt Lake City, UT 84119
800-825-4555
www.chisco.com
Never lose your glasses again; source for the eyeglass
necklaces.

Clover Needlecraft, Inc.
13438 Alondra Boulevard
Cerritos, California 90703-2315
800-233-1703
www.Clover-USA.com
Knitting and crocheting supplies.

DesignTech International, LLC
1 Viper Way
Vista, CA 92081
800-876-0800
www.DesignTech-Intl.com
Source for automotive accessories, such as remote start
systems and back-up alert devices.

Do Not Call Registry
888-382-1222
www.DoNotCall.gov
Stop unwanted telemarketing calls; register to be removed
from telemarketing lists.

DrivingComfort
P.O. Box 9036
Charlottesville, VA 22906
www.DrivingComfort.com
Source for vehicular accessories and gadgets to make
driving easier and more comfortable, such as special wide-
view automotive mirrors and portable jump starters.

Dynamic Living
95 W. Dudleytown Road
Bloomfield, CT 06002
888-940-0605
www.Dynamic-Living.com
Source for accessibility and adaptability items, including
offset hinges for wheelchair-accessible doorways, car
handles to make transfers to and from vehicles safer and
easier, and ULU knives and cutting boards.

ElderStore
6820 Meadowridge Court, Suite A-9
Alpharetta, GA 30005
888-833-8875
www.ElderStore.com
Source for many helpful products including seat belt extenders.

Fashionable Canes Co.
www.FasionableCanes.com
Fashionable and functional canes.

Forearm Forklift
www.ForearmForklift.com
Lifting straps to make lifting and carrying loads easier.

GNU Industries, Inc.
1919 NW 19th Street, Building 1A
Ft. Lauderdale, FL 33311
800-780-1409
www.CommandoAlarms.com
Source for security items, including the automatic car starter and keyless entry systems.

The Happy Company
26203 Production Avenue, Suite 4
Hayward, CA 94545
800-486-2896
www.TheHappyCompany.com

Health Craft Products, Inc.
2790 Fenton Road
Ottawa, ONT, Canada K1T 3T7
888-619-9992
www.HealthCraftProducts.com
Adaptability aids, including Smart Rail and the Super Pole System.

Independent Living Aids, Inc.
200 Robbins Lane
Jericho, NY 11753
800-537-2118
www.IndependentLiving.com
Source for deluxe edition and adaptive games.

Independent Living Centers
www.ilusa.com/links/ilcenters.htm
Source for information on independent living centers
across the country.

International Environmental Solutions, Inc./MEDFLO
2830 Scherer Drive North, Suite 310
St. Petersburg, FL 33716
800-972-8348
www.InternationalEnvironmentalSolutions.com
Source for the EZ-Flow water wand.

Keen Footwear Company
www.Keenfootwear.com
Sturdy, fashionable, comfortable supportive footwear.

Kerry Hills Farm
Surround Ewe™ Sleep Systems
N1237 Franklin Road
Oconomowoc, WI 53066
920-474-4503
www.KerryHillsFarm.com
Warm and comfortable wool underquilts, comforters,
and more.

Light on Call™
548 Sunrise Highway
West Babylon, NY 11704
631-587-7414
www.LightOnCall.com
A telephone-activated lighting system that can illuminate
your house with a phone call.

Maddak Inc.
661 Route 23 South
Wayne, NJ 07470
973-628-7600
www.maddak.com
Source for the Open-It Universal Opener, a multipurpose packaging and container opening tool and other helpful products.

MagnaJewelry
1924 Elmwood Avenue
Warwick, RI 02888
www.MagnaJewelry.com
Supplier of magnetic jewelry clasps that make putting on and taking off necklaces, bracelets, and other clasped jewelry easier.

Merrel Boot Company
www.Merrelboot.com
Supportive footwear.

Misty Mate, Inc.
955 North Fiesta Boulevard, Suite 1
Gilbert, AZ 85233
800-233-6478
www.MistyMate.com
Personal misters to keep you (and your houseplants) cool and hydrated.

Mix Match Shoes
236 East Knight Street
Eaton Rapids, MI 48827
888-726-9420
www.MixMatchShoes.com
Source for split-size shoes.

MOTUS Inc.
P.O. Box 872
Winnipeg, MAN, Canada R3P 2S1
204-489-8280
www.Motus.mb.ca
Ergonomic hand grips that can make any tool or utensil more user-friendly.

National Odd Shoe Exchange
P.O. Box 1120
Chandler, AZ 85244-1120
480-892-3484
www.OddShoe.org
Source for split-size and single shoes.

Nordstrom's
888-282-6060
www.Nordstrom.com
Source for split-size and single shoes.

North Coast Medical, Inc.
18305 Sutter Boulevard
Morgan Hill, CA 95037-2845
800-235-7054
www.BeAbleToDo.com
Household and hobby adaptability aids, including loop scissors to make cutting paper and crafts easier.

Nuance
1 Wayside Road
Burlington, MA 01803
781-565-5000
www.Nuance.com/NaturallySpeaking
Source for speech-recognition software, including Dragon Naturally Speaking.

OXO International
75 Ninth Avenue, 5th Floor
New York, NY 10011
800-545-4411

www.oxo.com
Great source for all sorts of kitchen gadgets and accessibility aids for cooks, featuring ergonomic and cushion-
handled kitchen utensils, spillproof mugs, and more.

Pacific Writing Instruments
650-355-2640
www.PenAgain.com
Source for ergonomic writing instruments.

Phil-E-Slide Inc.
9 Industrial Way
Atkinson, NH 03811
866-675-4338
www.Phil-e-Slide-US.com
Makers of the Phil-E-Slide disc that makes transfers to and
from vehicles easier and safer.

Planet Media Group
13515 Old Dock Road
Orlando, FL 32828
888-669-9697
www.HealthHistory.com
Source for handy Health and Medical History forms.

Products for Seniors
850 S Boulder Highway, Suite 171
Henderson NV 89015
800-566-6561
www.ProductsForSeniors.com
Home adaptability products, including lamp switch
enlargers, and touch-sensitive lamp converters

Remedy Interactive, Inc.
480 Gate Five Road, Suite 130
Sausalito, CA 94965
800-776-5545
www.RSIguard.com
Source for repetitive stress prevention software programs.

S&S® Worldwide
P.O. Box 513
75 Mill Street
Colchester, CT 06415
800-288-9941
www.ssww.com
Great source of games, hobby and craft supplies.

Sammons Preston
P.O. Box 5071
Bolingbrook, IL 60440-5071
800-323-5547

Service-dogs Internet Listserv
An online community of people with service dogs.

Silvert's
3280 Steeles Avenue West, Suite 18
Concord, ONT, Canada L4K 2Y2
800-387-7088
www.silverts.com
Pre-knotted ties and other clothing and accessories for
people with disabilities.

Smarthome™
16542 Millikan Avenue
Irvine, CA 92606
800-242 7329
www.Smarthome.com
Home adaptability aids, including keyless locks, telephone
intercom systems, and towel warming drawers.

Solutions
P.O. Box 6878
Portland, OR 97228
800-342-9988
www.Solutions.com
Home adaptability products, including suction cup
handles to use as temporary grab bars.

Sterling Service Dogs
3715 E. Fifteen Mile Road
Sterling Heights, MI 48310
586-977-9716
www.SterlingServiceDogs.org.
Information on service dogs.

Steven Enterprises
6053 Third Avenue South
Minneapolis, MN 55419
612-869-9794
www.Zackaroos.com
The source for Zackaroos elastic ties that turn any laced
shoe into a slip-on.

Superfeet Worldwide, Inc.
1419 Whitehorn Street
Ferndale, WA 98248
800-634-6618
www.Superfeet.com
Source for ergonomic and custom insoles.

TravelSox
The Summit South
300 Centerville Road, Suite 450S
Warwick, Rhode Island 02886
866-387-6762
wwwTravelSox.com
Comfortable, stylish support stockings for travel and
lounging.

Walking Cane Depot
www.WalkingCaneDepot.com
Fashionable and functional canes.

Walking Cane Store
www.TheWalkingCaneStore.com
Fashionable and functional canes.

Wannalancit Mills
650 Suffolk Street, Suite G-5
Lowell, MA 01854
800-811-8290
www.Wristies.com
Manufacturer of Wristies and Sleeves, warm half sleeves
for wrists and forearms.

Yaktrax, LLC
9221 Globe Center Drive
Morrisville, NC 27560
866-YAKTRAX (925-8729)
www.Yaktrax.com
Source for non-skid footwear.

Yoropen Corp.
www.YoropenCorp.com
Source for ergonomic writing instruments.

Index

walkers, 27–28
  accessories for, 28
  baby shoes, tennis balls for, 26
  nylon glides for, 26–27
  resources for, 28
  styles of, 26
  for transporting things, 26
walking. *See under* exercise
warmth. *See* staying warm
weekend getaways, 135–36
wheelchair, use of, 2, 129
windshield placard. *See* disabled
  parking privileges

winter chores, 67–68
wireless systems
  intercoms and, 39
  remote door entry system, 47
working smart, 9–10
work surface height, lowering of, 81
wrists. *See* hand and wrist care
writing things down. *See*
  communication; notes

YakTrax, 68, 71, 152
yard work, 63–64
yoga classes, 5, 121

About the Author

Arthritis: 300 Tips for Making Life Easier™

Shelley Peterman Schwarz and her husband Dave live in Madison, Wisconsin. They've been married since 1969, and are enjoying being the parents of two adult children, Jamie and Andrew, and grandparents to three little ones. Jamie and her husband David live and work in Chicago. They are parents of daughter, Jordan, and son, Matthew. Andrew and his wife, Ronit, live and work in Sacramento, CA. They are the parents of daughter, Gali.

At the time of her multiple sclerosis (MS) diagnosis in 1979, Shelley was working part-time as a teacher of the deaf. Two years later, due to the effects of progressive MS, she retired. In 1985, when a story she wrote appeared in *Inside MS*, the magazine of the National Multiple Sclerosis Society, a new career was born. Since then, Shelley has published more than 500 articles and received numerous awards including the Mother of the Year from the Wisconsin Chapter of the National MS Society, the Spirit of the American Woman Award from JC Penney, and she was named a Woman of Distinction by the YWCA.

Shelley is the host of the free, weekly *Making Life Easier* Internet radio program, available as a pod cast 24/7 at www.MakingLifeEasier.com. Shelley and her guests, who also live with chronic health problems, share personal stories, anecdotes, and lessons learned to help others discover and embrace their own strategies for coping with chronic illness.

Shelley's nationally syndicated, *Tips for Making Life Easier*™ column appears in numerous newspapers and magazines internationally including, *Momentum, Real Living with MS,* and *The Motivator*. Her tips are available on numerous web sites as well. In 1997, the National Arthritis Foundation, Inc., commissioned Shelley to write *250 Tips for Making Life with Arthritis Easier*, based on her "Making Life Easier" column. In this second edition, she has updated and revised the book and expanded its content to include more than *300 Tips for Making Life Easier*.™

Other books in the Tips for Making Life Easier™ series:

- *Dressing Tips and Clothing Resources for Making Life Easier* (Attainment Company, 2000)
- *Multiple Sclerosis: 300 Tips for Making Life Easier* (Demos Medical Publishing, 1999, 2005)
- *Parkinson's Disease: 300 Tips for Making Life Easier* (Demos Medical Publishing, 2002, 2005)
- *Organizing Your IEPs: Individualized Educational Plan for Special Education Students* (Attainment Company, 2005)
- *Memory Tips for Making Life Easier* (Attainment Company, 2006)

Shelley's words and stories also appear in the following books:

- *Child Development 11th Edition* (McGraw Hill, 2005)
- *Jewish Mothers Tell Their Stories: Acts of Love and Courage* (The Haworth Press, Inc., 2000)
- *A Second Chicken Soup for the Woman's Soul* (Health Communications, Inc., 1998)
- *Amazingly Simple Lessons We Learned After 50* (M. Evans and Co. Inc., 2001)

In 1995, Shelley self-published a book entitled, *Blooming Where You're Planted: Stories from the Heart*. The previously published essays chronicle her journey of change and self-discovery following her MS diagnosis. A professional speaker, Shelley's philosophy of life is to find solutions to whatever problems she faces and to help others do the same. Her motivational and inspirational keynotes and workshops help audiences see challenges in their lives as opportunities for personal growth. She shares her message of hope and teaches audiences how to "bloom wherever they're planted."

Visit www.MeetingLifesChallenges.com to contact Shelley, subscribe to her free Internet radio program and/or e-zine, to read her blog and personal essays, or to learn about her teleclasses and speaking appearances.